GUIDE TO

OVER·THE·COUNTER DRUGS, VITAMINS, AND NATURAL MEDICINES

D1286503

TIME
LIFE
BOOKS

ALEXANDRIA, VIRGINIA

TIME LIFE BOOKS

TIME-LIFE BOOKS IS A DIVISION OF TIME LIFE INC.

TIME LIFE INC.
President and CEO: GEORGE ARTANDI

TIME-LIFE CUSTOM PUBLISHING
Vice President and Publisher: TERRY NEWELL
Vice President of Sales and Marketing: NEIL LEVIN
Director of Special Sales: LIZ ZIEHL
Editor for Special Markets: ANNA BURGARD
Production Manager: CAROLYN BOUNDS
Quality Assurance Manager: JAMES KING
Special Contributors: RUTH THOMPSON, THUNDER HILL GRAPHICS
(PRODUCTION), CELIA BEATTIE (PROOFREADING), JUDY DAVIS (INDEXING)

THIS BOOK IS AN ADAPTATION OF THE TIME-LIFE EDITION
The Drug and Natural Medicine Advisor © 1997.

Director of Editorial Development: JENNIFER PEARCE
Editor: ROBERT SOMERVILLE
Deputy Editor: TINA S. MCDOWELL
Design Director: TINA TAYLOR
Text Editor: JIM WATSON
Associate Editors/Research and Writing: NANCY BLODGETT
(PRINCIPAL), STEPHANIE SUMMERS HENKE

The descriptions of medical conditions and treatments in this book should be considered as a reference source only; they are not intended to substitute for a healthcare practitioner's diagnosis, advice, and treatment. Always consult your physician or a qualified practitioner for proper medical care.

Before using any drug or natural medicine mentioned in this book, be sure to check the appropriate sections of this book and the product's label for any warnings or cautions. Keep in mind that herbal remedies are not as strictly regulated as drugs.

First printing. Printed in U.S.A.

TIME-LIFE is a trademark of Time Warner Inc. U.S.A.

Library of Congress Cataloging-in-Publication Data
Time-Life guide to over-the-counter drugs, vitamins, and natural medicines: more than 100 of the most common traditional and alternative medications, including: antibiotics, coenzyme Q10, decongestants, echinacea, folic acid, ibuprofen, St. Jonhn's wort.
p. cm
Includes index.
ISBN 0-7370-1103-3
1. Naturopathy—Encyclopedias.
2. Drugs, Nonprescription—Encyclopedias.
3. Alternative medicine—Encyclopedias.
I. Time-Life Books.
RZ433.T56 1998
615'.1—dc21   98-3426 CIP

Books published by Time-Life Custom Publishing are available at special bulk discount for promotional and premium use. Custom adaptations can also be created to meet your specific marketing goals. Call 1-800-323-5255.

Cover photographs courtesy of PhotoDisc
Cover design by Anna Burgard

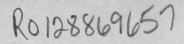

TABLE OF CONTENTS

INTRODUCTION

When you or someone you love is ill, the search for the right medication can be intimidating. You're faced with shelves full of choices. You want to know which drug is right for the specific symptoms you're trying to relieve, but may wonder: Will it interfere with any other drugs? What sort of side effects might occur? Is there an alternative remedy that could replace or supplement the more traditional medications?

This book is designed to give you access to vital information about the most common medications on the market, providing you with a base of knowledge to help you make informed, confident choices. More than 100 healing substances are listed alphabetically, from acetaminophen to ginkgo to zinc. Six types of therapies are included, from both the conventional and alternative, or natural, approaches to medicine. Each entry is designated by an icon indicating whether it is considered aromatherapy, Chinese medicine, a nutritional supplement, an over-the-counter/prescription drug (those that are available in both strengths), a vitamin or mineral, or a Western herb. (The Guide to Natural Therapies will introduce you to methods of healing that may be unfamiliar to you.)

Each entry provides both a broad overview of the medication and important specifics about its uses and effects, including a list of target ailments, possible side effects, precautions, and information about potential interactions with other drugs. Know what you're buying, and you'll be on the road to recovery quickly, and safely.

GUIDE TO
NATURAL THERAPIES

On the following pages you will find brief descriptions of the five forms of so-called natural therapies included in this book. Each of these introductions includes a general description of the therapy and the principles on which it is founded, followed by an explanation of the way each therapy's healing substances are prepared or applied. You should also take note of the Caution paragraph for each therapy. For three of the therapies, a separate box explains the licensing rules for practitioners and whether treatments are covered by insurance.

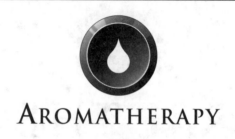

AROMATHERAPY

Aromatherapy is the therapeutic use of essential oils—concentrated, fragrant extracts of plants—to promote relaxation and help relieve various symptoms. Suppliers of aromatherapy oils extract them from specific parts of plants—the roots, bark, stalks, flowers, leaves, or fruit—by two methods: Distillation uses successive evaporation and condensation to pull the oils from the plants; cold-pressing squeezes rinds or peels through a machine to press out the oils. Users then administer the oils in several ways, generally by applying them to the skin or inhaling their scents.

Some practitioners believe the oils have both physical and ethereal (spiritual) qualities and effects. They assert that the oils work on the emotions because the nerves involved in the sense of smell are directly linked to the brain's limbic system, which governs emotion, and that the active components of the oils give them specific therapeutic value.

PREPARATIONS/TECHNIQUES

Essential oils may be applied externally and used in massage, or incorporated into compresses and ointments. They may also be inhaled or taken internally (orally, rectally, or vaginally). A common aromatherapy technique is to dilute the oils in a vegetable carrier oil, such as safflower or sweet almond oil, for an aromatherapy massage. Another way to use the oils is in an aromatic warm bath. You may also apply hot or cold compresses, creams, or lotions made from the oils directly to the skin.

CAUTION

Oils used in aromatherapy can have potentially serious side effects, including neurotoxicity and inducement of abortion as well as skin reactions, allergies, and liver damage. Overexposure to oils by inhalation can produce headache and fatigue. Consult a qualified healthcare practitioner before taking oils internally. Some oils, such as eucalyptus, lavender, myrrh, peppermint, and thyme, should never be taken internally.

LICENSED & INSURED?
Aromatherapy practitioners
are not licensed in the
United States today, although
licensed healthcare providers
may include aromatherapy
as one of their techniques.

CHINESE MEDICINE

Chinese medicine is an ancient system of healthcare that uses a variety of techniques, including herbal therapy, to treat disorders by restoring the balance of vital energies in the body. Unlike Western medicine, which tends to focus on specific parts of the body immediately affected by disease or injury, Chinese medicine takes a more global, holistic approach to healthcare, fashioning remedies to treat the entire body rather than just its component parts. Practitioners think of the human body not as a bundle of cells, bones, and tissues but rather as a complex system of interrelated processes. It is, they believe, a microcosm of the grand cosmic order, moved by the same rhythms and cycles that shape the natural world. At the core of Chinese medicine is the belief that disease is the result of disturbances in the flow of a bodily energy called chi or qi (pronounced "chee") or a lack of balance in the complementary states of yin (characterized by darkness and quiet) and yang (characterized by light and activity).

PREPARATIONS/TECHNIQUES

Chinese medicine recognizes more than 6,000 healing substances, although only a few hundred are currently in practical use. Herbs are grouped according to four basic properties, or "essences": hot, cold, warm, and cool. In general, practitioners choose plants for their ability to restore balance in individuals whose conditions are said to show signs of excessive heat or cold. Herbs are further categorized according to their "flavor": pungent, sour, sweet, bitter, or salty. An herb's taste indicates its action in the body, particularly on the movement and direction of chi.

Because many Chinese herbs work best when taken with others, practitioners almost always prescribe herbs in combination. Herbs are prepared in a variety of ways. Many are cooked and made into a soup or tea. In some cases the raw plants are ground into a powder, then combined with a binding agent and pressed into a pill. A number of herbs are cooked and processed into a powder and are then either mixed with warm water and swallowed or taken as capsules. Some herbs are made into pastes that are applied to the skin, while others are extracted in alcohol and used as tinctures.

CAUTION

Mixing herbs is an extremely tricky business. Certain Chinese herbs can be poisonous in large amounts, so you should always check with a qualified practitioner for the proper dosages. Some Chinese herbs, such as safflower flower, should be used with caution during pregnancy. Complex mixtures should be formulated only by a trained practitioner.

> ### LICENSED & INSURED?
> In the United States, practitioners of Chinese medicine usually operate under the title of "licensed" or "certified" acupuncturist. Few insurance providers reimburse patients for the cost of Chinese herbal treatments, although a number do cover acupuncture.

Herbal Therapy

Herbal medicines are prepared from a wide variety of plant materials—frequently the leaves, stems, roots, and bark but also the flowers, fruits, twigs, seeds, and exudates (material that oozes out, such as sap). They generally contain several biologically active ingredients and are used primarily for treating chronic or mild conditions, although on occasion they are employed as complementary or supportive therapy for acute and severe diseases.

Across the spectrum of alternative medicine, the use of herbs varies: Western herbology and Chinese medicine, for example, differ in the way practitioners diagnose diseases and prescribe herbal remedies. Naturopathic physicians, or those who use natural remedies rather than synthetic drugs, may use herbs from any of various systems. Entries in this book on herbs listed as Western herbs contain information based on Western herbological practices.

PREPARATIONS/TECHNIQUES

Herbs are available in various forms at health food stores and pharmacies, and many can be ordered by mail. Herbal remedies can be prepared at home in a variety of ways, using either fresh or dried ingredients. Herbal teas, or infusions, can be steeped to varying strengths. Roots, bark, or other plant parts can be simmered into strong solutions called decoctions. Honey or sugar can be added to infusions and decoctions to make syrups. You can also buy many herbal remedies over the counter in the form of pills, capsules, or powders, or in more concentrated liquid forms called extracts and tinctures. Certain herbs can be applied topically as creams or ointments, used as compresses, or applied directly to the skin as poultices.

CAUTION

Be especially careful when using herbs if you have allergies, are sensitive to drugs, are taking drugs for a chronic illness, or are younger than 12 or older than 65. To help minimize any adverse reactions, start with the lowest appropriate dose. Be aware that some herbs are toxic if taken incorrectly; comfrey, for example, can cause liver damage if taken in excessive amounts for too long a time.

In the United States today, herbal remedies are not regulated, and they come in unpredictable strengths because the amount of the active ingredients varies greatly. If you consistently develop nausea, diarrhea, or headache within two hours of taking an herb, discontinue its use immediately. Call your practitioner if the symptoms persist. Women who are pregnant or nursing are advised not to take medicinal amounts of herbs without first consulting a healthcare professional.

LICENSED & INSURED?

Naturopathic physicians are licensed on a state-by-state basis, and in some states their services are covered by medical insurance. However, clinical or medical herbalists are not licensed, and insurance companies usually do not provide coverage for their services.

NUTRITIONAL SUPPLEMENTS

Nutritional supplements are substances that are rich in essential nutrients or that contain ingredients helpful in the digestion or metabolism of food. In this book, the traditional definition of nutritional supplements as food or food by-products has been expanded to include a broader range of substances—such as hormones, amino acids, and plant or animal products—that are thought to provide certain health benefits.

Most people get all the nutrition they need from their diet. But sometimes the food we eat fails to deliver all the nutrients we require, perhaps as a result of disease, stress, poor eating habits, or a special medical condition. In such cases, supplements can help supply the missing ingredients and restore good health. Some of these products are taken for short periods to combat specific disorders. Others can be used long term—to ward off the effects of aging, for example, or to maintain good health and general wellness.

Because age impairs the body's ability to use nutrients effectively, the elderly often need to balance their diet with supplements. Other groups that may require supplemental nutrients include women who are pregnant, breast-feeding, or have excessive menstrual bleeding; heavy drinkers or smokers; strict vegetarians; and newborns.

PREPARATIONS/TECHNIQUES

Nutritional supplements are available in a variety of shapes and forms, including capsules, tablets, powders, liquids, flakes, gels, creams, wafers, and granules. Most are taken orally, although some are injected or applied to the skin. These products can be purchased at health food stores and at some pharmacies and grocery stores, or ordered through the mail. Potencies vary, and sometimes the potency is affected by temperature or the length of time the supplement sits on the shelf.

CAUTION

Some nutritional supplements can be poisonous if taken in large amounts. In other cases, excess amounts of one nutrient can actually reduce the body's supplies of another. Beware of combinations: Taken together, certain supplements can interact in the body and cause harmful effects. Because the quality of these products may vary considerably, you should always buy from a reputable source.

Be very skeptical of "miracle cures" and other wild claims about the effectiveness of nutritional supplements. Find out all you can about the product before using it, and remember that nothing takes the place of a balanced diet. You should also be aware that the efficacy and safety of some supplements listed in this book—such as EDTA, a synthetic amino acid used in chelation therapy—are under intense debate. Always consult a qualified practitioner before using any nutritional supplement.

VITAMINS AND MINERALS

A balanced diet is an essential part of a healthy lifestyle. Your body requires more than 40 nutrients for energy, growth, and tissue maintenance. In addition to carbohydrates, proteins, fats, and dietary fiber, the food you eat supplies the important micronutrients we call vitamins and minerals. They are needed only in trace amounts, but the absence or deficiency of just one vitamin or mineral can cause major illness.

Vitamin and mineral supplements figure in the dietary recommendations of many therapies. Although some vitamins, such as A and D, are fat soluble and can reach toxic levels in the body if they are not carefully monitored, others, such as vitamin C, are water soluble and are not stored; any bodily excess is usually excreted. Generally, vitamins and minerals are recommended for daily use as a preventive measure only, but some healthcare practitioners also suggest them as a treatment for specific ailments. Some such treatments are considered controversial, so it's best to check with your own practitioner.

PREPARATIONS/TECHNIQUES

Vitamin and mineral supplements often come in tablet form. Doses are measured by weight in milligrams (mg), or thousandths of a gram; in micrograms (mcg), or millionths of a gram; or in a universal standard known as international units (IU). The Food and Nutrition Board of the National Research Council, National Academy of Sciences, has determined a recommended dietary allowance (RDA)—also known as the recommended daily allowance—for many vitamins and minerals. Essential nutrients that do not yet have RDAs are assigned a safe and adequate daily intake or an estimated minimum daily requirement (EMDR). These values are listed in the vitamins and minerals entries in this book.

CAUTION

Always take supplements in moderation; they are safe in doses at or below RDAs, but higher doses may be harmful and should be taken only under the guidance of a doctor or registered dietitian. Be particularly cautious about fat-soluble vitamins such as A and D, excesses of which are harder for the body to handle.

A-TO-Z GUIDE TO
OVER-THE-COUNTER DRUGS, VITAMINS, AND NATURAL MEDICINES

SYMBOLS FOR SUBSTANCES:

 AROMATHERAPY

 OVER-THE-COUNTER AND PRESCRIPTION DRUGS

 CHINESE MEDICINE

 VITAMINS AND MINERALS

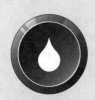 NUTRITIONAL SUPPLEMENTS

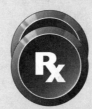 WESTERN HERBS

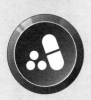 OVER-THE-COUNTER DRUGS

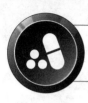

ACETAMINOPHEN

VITAL STATISTICS

DRUG CLASS
Analgesics

BRAND NAMES
Acetaminophen-only brands: Tylenol, Tylenol Extra Strength
Acetaminophen-containing combinations for colds: Chlor-Trimeton Allergy-Sinus Headache Caplets, Comtrex, Contac, Drixoral, TheraFlu, Triaminic Sore Throat Formula, Tylenol in various forms, Vicks DayQuil Liquid or LiquiCaps, Vicks NyQuil
Combinations for pain: Excedrin Extra-Strength, Tylenol in various forms
Combinations for sinus problems: Sinutab
Combinations for sleep: Excedrin PM

OTHER DRUGS IN THIS CLASS
aspirin, caffeine (as an adjunct treatment), methyl salicylate, nonsteroidal anti-inflammatory drugs (NSAIDs), opioid analgesics

GENERAL DESCRIPTION
A pain reliever as well as a fever reducer, acetaminophen is a good alternative to aspirin, particularly for people who are allergic to aspirin. One drawback is that acetaminophen does not reduce inflammation, so it is not effective for such conditions as swelling, redness, or menstrual cramps. If you seek relief from inflammation, try aspirin or a nonsteroidal anti-inflammatory drug.

PRECAUTIONS

SPECIAL INFORMATION
- Acetaminophen can cause or exacerbate liver problems, so you should avoid alcoholic beverages when taking this drug. If you are too sick to eat, even moderate overdoses of acetaminophen can cause serious liver damage, possibly leading to convulsions, coma, and death. If you already have liver disease, use acetaminophen with caution, preferably under a doctor's supervision.
- Don't take more than the recommended dose. Persistent pain or high fever may indicate serious illness. If pain persists for more than 10 days or fever lasts for three days, contact your physician.
- If an overdose occurs, seek emergency help. Possible symptoms of overdose include nausea, vomiting, increased sweating, loss of appetite, and abdominal pain, although in some cases there are no symptoms. Treatment must start within 24 hours to prevent severe liver (and possible kidney) damage.
- To avoid involuntary overdose, be careful when combining this drug with other medications that contain acetaminophen. Read labels carefully.

Acetaminophen

POSSIBLE INTERACTIONS

Alcohol: risk of liver damage.

Anticoagulants (oral): if acetaminophen is taken regularly and in high doses, this combination can lead to an increased anticoagulant effect.

Aspartame: possibly hazardous for phenylketonuria patients.

Aspirin: risk of increased side effects of both drugs when combination is taken over a long period.

Barbiturates (except butalbital): reduced acetaminophen effect. Taking too much acetaminophen in combination with barbiturates also increases the risk of liver damage.

Isoniazid: risk of liver damage.

Nonsteroidal anti-inflammatory drugs (NSAIDs): risk of increased side effects of either drug when combination is taken over a long period.

Zidovudine (AZT): increased blood levels of zidovudine and risk of serious side effects.

TARGET AILMENTS

Fever

Headaches, muscle aches, pain, or injuries

SIDE EFFECTS

SERIOUS

- Hypersensitivity reaction (rash, hives, itching)
- Kidney damage (lower-back pain, sudden reduction in urine output)
- Liver damage (pain or swelling in the upper abdominal area) or hepatitis (jaundice)
- Blood disorder (unusual sore throat or fever)
- Anemia (unusual fatigue)
- Platelet disorder (unusual bruising or bleeding; black, tarry stools; bloody or cloudy urine)

(RARE, IF TAKEN IN RECOMMENDED DOSES): IF YOU NOTICE ANY OF THESE SYMPTOMS, DISCONTINUE USE AND CALL YOUR DOCTOR IMMEDIATELY.

ALOE

LATIN NAME
Aloe barbadensis

VITAL STATISTICS

GENERAL DESCRIPTION

This tropical herb yields two therapeutic substances. The first, a translucent gel, works externally to relieve minor burns, skin irritations, and infections; taken internally, aloe gel relieves stomach disorders. It is used as a beauty aid and moisturizer because it contains polysaccharides, which act as emollients to soothe, soften, and protect the skin.

The second remedy contained in the aloe plant is a bitter yellow juice known as latex, which acts as a powerful laxative.

PREPARATIONS
Over the counter:
Available as powder, fluidextract, powdered capsules, bottled gel, or latex tablets.

At home:
EYEWASH: Dissolve ½ tsp powdered aloe gel in 1 cup water. Add 1 tsp boric acid to accelerate healing. Pour the solution through a coffee filter before applying to the eyes.
BATH: Add 1 to 2 cups aloe gel to a warm bath to relieve sunburn or skin lesions.
COMBINATIONS: Use aloe gel with wheat-germ oil and safflower flower to reduce bruising. Consult a practitioner for the dosage appropriate for you and the ailment being treated.

PRECAUTIONS

☠ WARNING
Do not exceed the recommended dose of aloe latex. Pregnant and nursing women should not take aloe internally.

SPECIAL INFORMATION
If you have a gastrointestinal illness, take aloe internally only in consultation with an herbalist or a licensed healthcare professional.

POSSIBLE INTERACTIONS
Combining aloe with other herbs may necessitate a lower dosage.

SIDE EFFECTS

NOT SERIOUS
- Allergic dermatitis
- Intestinal cramps
- Diarrhea

TRY A LOWER DOSAGE OR STOP USING THE PRODUCT.

TARGET AILMENTS

Take aloe gel internally for:

Digestive disorders
Gastritis
Stomach ulcers

Use aloe latex internally for:

Constipation

Use aloe gel externally for:

Minor burns; sunburn
Infection in wounds
Insect bites
Acne; skin irritations
Bruising
Chickenpox
Poison ivy
Irritated eyes

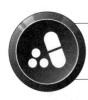

ALUMINUM HYDROXIDE

Upset stomach; heartburn

Acid indigestion; sour stomach

Ulcers

VITAL STATISTICS

DRUG CLASS
Antacids

BRAND NAMES
Gaviscon; some types of Maalox and Mylanta

OTHER DRUGS IN THIS CLASS
calcium carbonate, magnesium carbonate, magnesium hydroxide, sodium bicarbonate and citric acid

GENERAL DESCRIPTION
Aluminum hydroxide is an aluminum-containing antacid used to relieve upset and sour stomach, heartburn, acid indigestion, and some types of ulcers. It is most effective when taken on an empty stomach. The most common adverse effect of aluminum hydroxide is constipation. See Antacids for more information, including facts about possible drug interactions and additional special information.

PRECAUTIONS

SPECIAL INFORMATION
- Check with your doctor before taking aluminum hydroxide if you are on kidney dialysis; aluminum toxicity could result.
- Because they can affect the rate of absorption of other drugs, antacids should not be taken within one to two hours of many other oral medications. Ask your doctor or pharmacist for guidance.
- Notify your doctor if you develop symptoms such as black, tarry stools or vomit the consistency of coffee grounds. These are indications of bleeding in the stomach or intestines.

SIDE EFFECTS

NOT SERIOUS
- Mild constipation
- Laxative effect or diarrhea
- Chalky taste in the mouth
- Stomach cramps, nausea, or vomiting
- Belching
- Flatulence
- White specks in the stool

CALL YOUR DOCTOR IF THESE PROBLEMS PERSIST.

SERIOUS
- Swelling of the wrist, foot, or lower leg
- Bone pain
- Severe constipation
- Dizziness
- Mood changes
- Muscle pain, weakness, or twitching
- Nervousness or restlessness
- Slow breathing
- Irregular heartbeat
- Fatigue
- Pain upon urinating or frequent need to urinate
- Change in appetite

CONTACT YOUR DOCTOR IMMEDIATELY.

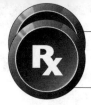

ANALGESICS

VITAL STATISTICS

GENERIC NAMES
acetaminophen, aspirin; caffeine (adjunct therapy); methyl salicylate (topical analgesic)

Nonsteroidal Anti-Inflammatory Drugs (NSAIDs): diclofenac, etodolac, flurbiprofen, ibuprofen, ketoprofen, ketorolac, nabumetone, naproxen, oxaprozin

Opioid Analgesics: codeine, hydrocodone, oxycodone, propoxyphene, tramadol

GENERAL DESCRIPTION
Analgesics are drugs that relieve pain. Some, such as the opioid analgesics, offer relief by affecting the brain and nervous system; these drugs are sometimes called narcotics because they can cause physical and psychological dependence. Nonnarcotic pain relievers, on the other hand, act at the site of the pain, usually by relieving inflammation. Sometimes two or more analgesics are combined to increase the effectiveness or the range of their action.

Aspirin, among the most popular of all over-the-counter pain relievers, is used to treat headache, arthritis, muscle aches, and minor injuries. It is also taken to suppress fever, reduce inflammation, and lower the risk of heart attack. Acetaminophen, widely used to relieve pain and reduce fever, is a good alternative to aspirin, although acetaminophen does not reduce inflammation. The opioid analgesic codeine helps control coughing and is often prescribed along with aspirin or acetaminophen for moderate pain relief. Ibuprofen, an over-the-counter drug used to relieve the pain of headaches, menstrual cramps, muscle aches, and certain types of arthritis, also reduces inflammation and fever.

Analgesics have side effects that depend on their mode of action and also on individual response. Some can cause drowsiness or a severe allergic reaction, while others may affect the digestive system or blood vessels.

PRECAUTIONS

☠ WARNING
Do not give aspirin to children or teenagers with fevers. Aspirin can provoke a potentially fatal liver inflammation called Reye's syndrome in young people if the drug is used to treat a fever or viral infection such as chickenpox or influenza.

TARGET AILMENTS
Fever
Headaches
Muscle and joint aches
Pain, especially from injuries or surgery
Inflammation associated with menstrual cramps, arthritis, bursitis, and other conditions

ANESTHETICS

VITAL STATISTICS

GENERIC NAMES
benzocaine, dyclonine, pramoxine

GENERAL DESCRIPTION
Over-the-counter anesthetics are topical drugs used to relieve pain and discomfort by blocking the initiation and conduction of nerve impulses to the brain. They are used on all body surfaces and in easily accessible areas inside the body, such as the mouth and esophagus.

Although the most commonly used over-the-counter anesthetics are for mouth pain, the drugs are also found in preparations used to treat minor burns, sunburn, and rectal pain (from hemorrhoids), and to aid in medical examinations and minor surgical procedures. These medications have relatively few side effects except when used excessively, which results in their absorption into the bloodstream, or when they trigger an allergic or hypersensitivity reaction.

PRECAUTIONS

SPECIAL INFORMATION
- Before using dyclonine or pramoxine, consult your doctor if you are pregnant or nursing or have heart disease, high blood pressure, thyroid disease, or diabetes.
- Some anesthetic preparations can be applied to the mouth or throat; others, including those that contain pramoxine, are for external application only. Read labels carefully.

TARGET AILMENTS

Canker sores (benzocaine, dyclonine)

Mouth or gum injury (benzocaine, dyclonine)

Toothache (benzocaine, dyclonine)

Cold sores; minor burns (pramoxine)

Uncomplicated hemorrhoidal itching and pain (pramoxine)

SIDE EFFECTS

NOT SERIOUS
- Burning sensation in the eyes (pramoxine)
- Irritation or stinging of mucous membranes

CALL YOUR DOCTOR IF THESE EFFECTS CONTINUE.

SERIOUS
- Allergic skin reactions, burning, stinging, or hive-like swelling
- Cardiovascular effects including irregular heartbeat, low blood pressure, fainting
- Overdose effects, including nervousness, dizziness, tremors, seizures, blurred vision, ringing in the ears, respiratory depression

CALL YOUR DOCTOR RIGHT AWAY.

ANTACIDS

VITAL STATISTICS

GENERIC NAMES
aluminum hydroxide, calcium carbonate, magnesium carbonate, magnesium hydroxide, sodium bicarbonate and citric acid

GENERAL DESCRIPTION
Antacids relieve the occasional unpleasant symptoms that accompany heartburn, acid indigestion, and "sour" stomach. The drugs work to neutralize excess gastric acid in the stomach, and as a result they help to heal and reduce the pain of ulcers. Antacids are most effective when taken on an empty stomach.

Many popular antacid preparations are combinations of different generic drugs. These combination antacids, such as aluminum and magnesium or calcium and magnesium, have the advantage of offsetting either constipation or diarrhea.

Taken regularly over a long period of time, some calcium-containing antacids may help prevent osteoporosis and other conditions associated with calcium deficiency.

PRECAUTIONS

SPECIAL INFORMATION
- Except under special circumstances determined by your doctor, antacids should not be used if you have impaired renal function or if you have high levels of calcium in your blood, a condition known as hypercalcemia.
- If you have any of the following conditions, you and your doctor will have to weigh the benefits and risks of taking the different types of antacids: symptoms of appendicitis; gastrointestinal or rectal bleeding of undiagnosed cause; intestinal obstruction; sensitivity to aluminum, calcium, magnesium, simethicone, or sodium bicarbonate medications.
- Before taking antacids, check with your doctor if you have had a colostomy or ileostomy, or if you have any of the following: cirrhosis, congestive heart failure, edema, colitis, diverticulitis, diarrhea, constipation or fecal impaction, hemorrhoids, sarcoidosis (a rare disease manifested by lesions in the skin, eyes, lungs, and lymph nodes), or hypophosphatemia (abnormally low concentrations of phosphates in the blood).

ANTACIDS

- Children under the age of six should not take antacids without a doctor's approval.
- Notify your doctor if you develop symptoms such as black, tarry stools or vomit the consistency of coffee grounds. These are indications of bleeding in the stomach or intestines.
- Although antacids are considered safe if taken in low doses and for short periods (under two weeks), pregnant and nursing women should consult a doctor first; antacids containing sodium may increase fluid retention.
- Any long-term antacid therapy—such as the treatment of ulcers—should be administered by a doctor.
- Because they can affect the rate of absorption of other drugs, antacids should not be taken within one to two hours of many other oral medications. Ask your doctor or pharmacist for guidance.
- If taken for any length of time, antacids can have a rebound effect that worsens your symptoms when you stop taking the medication.
- Calcium carbonate and sodium bicarbonate antacids can cause milk-alkali syndrome, which is characterized by headaches, nausea, irritability, and weakness. In time, milk-alkali syndrome can lead to kidney disease or failure.

POSSIBLE INTERACTIONS

Staggering medication times is one way to avoid undesirable drug interactions.

Anticholinergics, digoxin, phenothiazines, quinidine, warfarin: antacids are known to interfere with the effectiveness of these drugs.

Aspirin and other salicylates: antacids may increase excretion of these drugs, lessening their effectiveness. Do not take aspirin or other salicylates within three to four hours of antacids.

Cellulose sodium phosphate: the ability of this drug to reduce hypercalciuria (excretion of abnormally large amounts of calcium in the urine) may be lessened when it is taken with calcium antacids.

Enteric-coated medications: antacids may cause the enteric coating to dissolve too rapidly, resulting in gastric irritation. Do not take these medications within one to two hours of antacids.

Iron: decreased iron absorption. Space doses of iron and antacids as far apart as possible (12 hours).

Isoniazid (oral): absorption of this antituber-

TARGET AILMENTS
Upset stomach
Heartburn
Acid indigestion
Sour stomach
Ulcers
Calcium deficiency (calcium carbonate)

CONTINUED

ANTACIDS

cular drug may be delayed and decreased when taken with antacids.

Ketoconazole (antifungal drug): absorption of ketoconazole may be reduced when taken within three hours of antacids.

Mecamylamine: antacids may prolong the effects of this high blood pressure drug. Do not take mecamylamine with antacids.

Methenamine: this drug, used to treat urinary tract infections, may be less effective when taken with antacids.

Phenytoin should not be taken within two to three hours of antacids, since antacids may decrease absorption of this seizure-control drug.

Quinolones: reduced effectiveness of quinolones and fluoroquinolones.

Sodium polystyrene sulfonate (a cholesterol-reducing drug): risk of kidney failure and alkalosis.

Tetracycline (antibiotic): decreased absorption of tetracycline; do not take this drug within three to four hours of antacids.

Vitamin D: if taken concurrently with antacids containing either magnesium or calcium, vitamin D can result in abnormally large amounts of either mineral in the blood.

SIDE EFFECTS

NOT SERIOUS

- Mild constipation
- Laxative effect or diarrhea
- Chalky taste in the mouth
- Stomach cramps, nausea, or vomiting
- Belching
- Flatulence
- White specks in the stool

CALL YOUR DOCTOR IF THESE PROBLEMS PERSIST.

SERIOUS

- Swelling of the wrist, foot, or lower leg
- Bone pain
- Severe constipation
- Dizziness
- Mood changes
- Muscle pain, weakness, or twitching
- Nervousness or restlessness
- Slow breathing
- Irregular heartbeat
- Fatigue
- Pain upon urinating or frequent need to urinate

CONTACT YOUR DOCTOR IMMEDIATELY.

ANTIBIOTICS

VITAL STATISTICS

GENERIC NAMES
clindamycin, nitrofurantoin
Carbacephems: loracarbef
Cephalosporins: cefaclor, cefadroxil, cefalexin
hydrochloride, cefixime, cefprozil, cefti-
buten, cefuroxime, cephalexin
Erythromycins: azithromycin, clarithromycin,
erythromycin
Fluoroquinolones: ciprofloxacin, ofloxacin
Ophthalmic Antibiotics: erythromycin,
tobramycin
Penicillins: amoxicillin, amoxicillin and
clavulanate, ampicillin, penicillin V
Sulfonamides in Combination: sulfamethoxa-
zole and trimethoprim
Tetracyclines: doxycycline, tetracycline
Topical Antibiotics: bacitracin, chlorhexidine,
mupirocin, neomycin, polymyxin B

TARGET AILMENTS
Bacterial infections, including
those of the respiratory tract,
urinary tract, skin, and eyes

GENERAL DESCRIPTION
Antibiotics are a large class of drugs used
against bacterial infections, such as strep
throat, otitis media, and other infections of
the respiratory tract, eyes, skin, and other
organs. Bactericidal antibiotics kill bacteria by
attacking bacterial cell walls. Bacteriostatic
antibiotics prevent bacteria from reproducing,
thus enabling the body's defenses to over-
come the infection. Antibiotics are not effective against fungal infections or against viruses, such as those that cause colds.

Because antibiotics target bacteria and
not fungi, the drugs can disturb the body's
normal balance of fungi and bacteria. This imbalance may be manifested as a fungal superinfection, such as a yeast infection, or in
symptoms of diarrhea or gastrointestinal dis-
turbance. To help restore your body's normal
bacteria, some doctors recommend eating yogurt that contains *Lactobacillus acidophilus*
culture or taking acidophilus tablets during
antibiotic therapy and for a week afterward.

PRECAUTIONS

SPECIAL INFORMATION
To prevent reinfection, take the full course of
your prescription, even if you feel better before you've taken all the medicine.

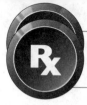

ANTIFUNGAL DRUGS

VITAL STATISTICS

GENERIC NAMES

Rx: clotrimazole, fluconazole, ketoconazole, miconazole, terconazole
OTC: clotrimazole, miconazole, tolnaftate, undecylenate

GENERAL DESCRIPTION

Antifungal drugs are used to treat a wide variety of conditions, including fungal infections of the skin, lungs, mouth, groin, hands, feet, and nails. Ringworm infections, including athlete's foot and jock itch, are among the best-known groups of skin disorders for which these drugs are used. Some antifungal medications are also used to treat yeast infections of the mouth (oral thrush); skin folds and hands; urethra, penis and foreskin (balanitis); and vagina.

Antifungal drugs work in different ways to interfere with the growth and reproduction of fungal cells or, in strong concentrations, to destroy fungal cells. These medications can be topical, vaginal, or systemic (acting throughout the body) and are available as creams, suppositories, lotions, powders, sprays, shampoos, lozenges, and oral tablets.

Topical lotions, creams, powders, and sprays are applied directly to the skin to treat fungal skin infections. Because they are massaged into the skin, creams and ointments are more effective than sprays and powders for the treatment of skin infections. Spray and powder forms of antifungal medications are effective in preventing fungal skin infections.

Vaginal antifungal creams and suppositories are inserted directly into the vagina, usually at bedtime, for a period of three to seven days.

Systemic antifungal medications (ketoconazole) are available in oral suspension and tablet form. They are used to treat a variety of disorders, including pneumonia and urinary tract infections.

See Vaginal Antifungal Drugs for information about a subclass of medications commonly used to treat vaginal yeast infections.

TARGET AILMENTS

Yeast infections (candidiasis) of the vulva and vagina, mouth, skin, hands, and internal organs

Ringworm (tinea) of the body, scalp, nails, hands, feet (athlete's foot), and groin (jock itch)

Tinea versicolor, a ringworm infection that produces white-brown patches on the skin

Fungal diseases of the lungs

Fungal skin infections (topical)

Seborrheic dermatitis

Dandruff

ANTIFUNGAL DRUGS

SPECIAL INFORMATION

- Do not use any topical antifungal medications if you have had an allergic reaction to another drug of this type. Check first with your physician or pharmacist.
- Although ringworm medications are available in over-the-counter form, be sure your condition has been correctly diagnosed before treating it yourself.
- Be sure to wash and thoroughly dry the infected area before using creams and ointments to treat skin infections.
- It is very important to medicate the entire area when treating an active fungal infection. If you have athlete's foot, for example, you need to apply the medication between all toes, to the skin around each toenail, and to the sole of the foot. Both feet should be treated with the same thorough care.
- Pregnant and nursing women should avoid antifungal medications, unless administered under a doctor's care.
- Because fungi thrive in moist conditions, avoid tight-fitting shoes and underwear made with synthetic fibers during treatment; wear cotton underwear instead.

POSSIBLE INTERACTIONS

No interactions are expected with most topical and vaginal forms of antifungal drugs.

SIDE EFFECTS

NOT SERIOUS

- Mild skin irritation in the infected area
- Headache
- Drowsiness
- Dizziness
- Nausea or vomiting
- Stomach pain
- Constipation or diarrhea

CALL YOUR DOCTOR IF THESE SIDE EFFECTS PERSIST OR BECOME BOTHERSOME.

SERIOUS

- Allergic skin reactions, such as a rash or hives (topical preparations)
- Redness, stinging, burning, or itching of the genitals; abdominal cramps or menstrual irregularities; or itching and burning of a sexual partner's penis (vaginal preparations)

CALL YOUR DOCTOR IF YOU EXPERIENCE ANY OF THESE SIDE EFFECTS.

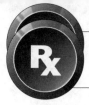

ANTIHISTAMINES

VITAL STATISTICS

GENERIC NAMES
Rx: astemizole, cetirizine, diphenhydramine, fexofenadine, loratadine, promethazine, terfenadine
OTC: brompheniramine, chlorpheniramine, clemastine, dexbrompheniramine, diphenhydramine, doxylamine, triprolidine

BRAND NAMES
Rx brands:
Allegra (fexofenadine); Benadryl (diphenhydramine); Claritin, Claritin-D 12 Hour (loratadine); Hismanal (astemizole); Phenergan (promethazine); Seldane, Seldane-D (terfenadine); Zyrtec (cetirizine)

OTC brands:
- Dimetapp (brompheniramine)
- Alka-Seltzer Plus Cold Medicine, Children's Tylenol Cold Multi-Symptom, Children's Tylenol Cold Plus Cough, Chlor-Trimeton, Comtrex Multi-Symptom Cold Reliever, TheraFlu, Triaminic Nite Light, Triaminic Syrup, Triaminicol Multi-Symptom Relief, Tylenol Allergy Sinus, Tylenol Cold Multi-Symptom Formula (chlorpheniramine)
- Tavist-D (clemastine)
- Drixoral Cold and Flu, Drixoral Cold and Allergy (dexbrompheniramine)
- Benadryl, Excedrin PM, Tylenol Allergy Sinus Night Time Medication, Tylenol Cold Night Time Medication Liquid, Tylenol Flu Night Time, Tylenol PM, Unisom (diphenhydramine)
- NyQuil (doxylamine)
- Actifed (triprolidine)

GENERAL DESCRIPTION
Antihistamines block the action of histamine, a natural substance the body releases when fighting infection and in allergic reactions; histamine causes the runny nose, watery eyes, congestion, and hives or itching associated with allergies. Antihistamines are used primarily to relieve the symptoms of allergies and colds, although they cannot cure the underlying conditions. Since a common side effect of the older antihistamines is drowsiness, some are used as sleeping aids. The newer antihistamines—astemizole, fexofenadine, loratadine, and terfenadine—are less likely to cause drowsiness.

Antihistamines

PRECAUTIONS

SPECIAL INFORMATION

- Antihistamines are considered unsafe for women who are pregnant or nursing.
- Many antihistamines are considered unsafe for children under the age of 12. Some are appropriate if the child's dosage is determined by a physician or, in the case of OTC drugs, printed on the label. Children may be more susceptible to side effects than adults. Their reactions to a high dose are different too; while adults may experience sedation and lethargy, children are more likely to become jittery and nervous, and may have trouble sleeping.
- To avoid drowsiness, take less of the drug or try another antihistamine. Some antihistamines, such as loratadine, do not cause drowsiness, and over time you may develop a partial tolerance to the drugs that do.
- If you are taking an antihistamine that causes drowsiness, avoid driving or operating machinery until you know how the drug affects you.
- Some antihistamines, especially astemizole, loratadine, and terfenadine, may cause palpitations, fainting, cardiac arrest, or other serious heart disorders if taken in dosages higher than those recommended. Follow the dosage instructions carefully.
- If antihistamines give you an upset stomach, nausea, diarrhea, or other gastrointestinal problems, take the pills with meals or with milk.
- Check with your doctor before using antihistamines if you have asthma, narrow-angle glaucoma, an enlarged prostate, a stomach ulcer, a bladder obstruction, heart disease, or liver disease; the drugs may exacerbate these conditions.
- The Food and Drug Administration recently announced its intention to withdraw approval of terfenadine; it considers the drug fexofenadine to be a safer alternative, with essentially the same benefits. Talk with your doctor about the best medication for you.

TARGET AILMENTS

Nasal and respiratory allergies (seasonal and nonseasonal), including hay fever

Common cold (although antihistamines alone are not effective for most cold symptoms)

Allergic skin reactions (to poison ivy and insect bites, for example)

Insomnia (except astemizole, fexofenadine, loratadine, and terfenadine)

Motion sickness (diphenhydramine and promethazine)

CONTINUED

ANTIHISTAMINES

POSSIBLE INTERACTIONS

Alcohol: likely to increase the sedative effects of certain antihistamines; do not drink when you take these drugs.

Antianxiety drugs; barbiturates or other sedatives: do not take with antihistamines, as the combination may result in excessive sedation.

Clarithromycin, erythromycin, itraconazole, and ketoconazole: may interfere with the body's metabolism of astemizole, loratadine, or terfenadine and cause life-threatening cardiac problems. WARNING: Do not combine these drugs with astemizole, loratadine, or terfenadine.

MAO inhibitors: can cause hypotension and dryness of the respiratory passages when taken with antihistamines. Do not combine these drugs with antihistamines.

SIDE EFFECTS

NOT SERIOUS

- Drowsiness in varying degrees—avoid driving or operating machinery until you know how the antihistamine you are taking affects you
- Dizziness, weakness, and slower movement and reaction time
- Dryness of the mouth, nose, or throat
- Nervousness, restlessness, and insomnia, especially in children
- Upset stomach, nausea, and change in bowel habits

CALL YOUR DOCTOR IF THESE SYMPTOMS CONTINUE OR BECOME BOTHERSOME.

SERIOUS

- Fainting or irregular heart rhythms caused by astemizole, loratadine, and terfenadine (rare)

CALL YOUR DOCTOR IMMEDIATELY IF YOU NOTICE ANY CHANGE IN YOUR HEARTBEAT.

- Itchiness, rash, or inflammation caused by topical antihistamines (uncommon)

IF YOU THINK ANTIHISTAMINES ARE CAUSING THESE SYMPTOMS, DISCONTINUE USE AND TELL YOUR DOCTOR.

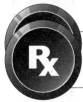

ANTIULCER DRUGS

VITAL STATISTICS

GENERIC NAMES
lansoprazole, omeprazole, sucralfate
Histamine H$_2$ blockers: cimetidine, famotidine, nizatidine, ranitidine

GENERAL DESCRIPTION
Antiulcer drugs are used to treat disorders associated with the overproduction of stomach acid, such as gastritis, gastroesophageal reflux, multiple endocrine neoplasia, Zollinger-Ellison syndrome, and, most commonly, ulcers of the stomach and duodenum (first portion of the small intestine). In general, antiulcer drugs work by inhibiting the production of the stomach's digestive juices, most notably hydrochloric acid and the digestive enzyme pepsin. Individual drugs achieve this effect in different ways.

Medications among the subclass of antiulcer drugs known as histamine H$_2$ blockers (including cimetidine, famotidine, nizatidine, and ranitidine) block the stomach's response to the chemical compound histamine, thereby reducing the secretion of hydrochloric acid. The drugs lansoprazole and omeprazole reduce the production of hydrochloric acid by inhibiting the action of enzymes in the acid-producing cells of the stomach lining. The exact mechanism of sucralfate is not completely understood, but the drug is believed to inhibit the digestive action of pepsin. It may also form a coating over stomach and duodenal ulcers, protecting them from the erosive effect of hydrochloric acid.

Antacids and antibiotics may also be used to treat ulcers.

PRECAUTIONS

☠ WARNING
Rare or infrequent side effects that are not serious include dizziness, lightheadedness, constipation, mild drowsiness, headache, mild diarrhea, skin rash, itching or other skin problems, muscle or joint pain, hair loss, temporary impotence and decreased libido, breast enlargement and tenderness (in women or men), abdominal pain, heartburn, indigestion, nausea, gas, appetite loss, dry mouth or skin, insomnia, depression, and anxiety. Call your doctor if these effects persist or become bothersome.

TARGET AILMENTS

Duodenal ulcer

Gastric ulcer

Upper gastrointestinal bleeding associated with gastric ulcer or duodenal ulcer, or with gastritis

Zollinger-Ellison syndrome, multiple endocrine neoplasia, and other conditions characterized by an overproduction of stomach acid

Gastroesophageal reflux

Gastrointestinal symptoms associated with the use of nonsteroidal anti-inflammatory drugs (NSAIDs) and aspirin

Heartburn or acid indigestion (OTC formulas)

CONTINUED

ANTIULCER DRUGS

SPECIAL INFORMATION

- Do not take these medications if you have had an allergic reaction or any unusual reactions to an antiulcer drug in the past.
- The side effects of the various antiulcer medications differ from drug to drug.
- Avoid antiulcer drugs if you are pregnant or nursing.
- Be sure to inform your doctor if you have any other medical problems, especially kidney or liver disease or any disease that causes obstruction of the gastrointestinal tract.
- Antiulcer drugs can interfere with the accuracy of some laboratory tests. Be sure to tell the person giving you a lab test that you are taking one of these drugs.
- Remember that some medications—such as aspirin and nonsteroidal anti-inflammatory drugs (NSAIDs)—and certain foods and drinks, including citrus products and beverages that are carbonated, alcoholic, or caffeinated, may irritate your stomach and make your problem worse.
- Check with your doctor before using antacids concurrently with an antiulcer drug.

POSSIBLE INTERACTIONS

Antiulcer drugs interact with many prescription and over-the-counter medications, some of which are listed below. Be sure to inform your doctor of any other drugs you may be taking.

Alcohol, caffeine, carbonated drinks, citrus foods, tobacco: may stimulate secretion of stomach acid and slow ulcer recovery rate; drinking alcoholic beverages while taking a histamine H_2 blocker may also increase blood levels of alcohol.

Alprazolam, carbamazepine, diazepam, digitalis preparations, glipizide, metoprolol, oral anticoagulants (including aspirin, dipyridamole, heparin): histamine H_2 blockers may increase the effects and possibly the toxicity of these drugs.

Aluminum-containing antidiarrheal drugs, aspirin buffered with aluminum, and aluminum-containing vaginal douches: sucralfate may increase the absorption of aluminum into the body, possibly to toxic levels.

Antacids: reduced effects of antiulcer drugs. Sometimes switching to another type of antacid or taking the antacid and the antiulcer drug at different times of the day can eliminate this problem. Consult your doctor. Avoid aluminum-containing antacids while taking sucralfate; the combination may lead to weakening of the bones and other symptoms of aluminum toxicity.

Aspirin: stomach irritation; increased effect of aspirin if large doses of aspirin are taken with nizatidine.

Cimetidine, ciprofloxacin, digoxin, ofloxacin, phenytoin, ranitidine, tetracycline, theophylline, warfarin: sucralfate may decrease the effectiveness of these drugs; omeprazole may increase the effects of phenytoin and warfarin.

Enteric-coated tablets: changes in stomach acidity may cause these drugs to dissolve prematurely in the stomach; avoid taking enteric-coated medications with cimetidine, famotidine, and nizatidine.

Iron: absorption of iron into the body may be inhibited by omeprazole.

Itraconazole and ketoconazole: omeprazole and histamine H_2 blockers may inhibit the absorption of these drugs into the body.

Vitamins A, D, E, and K: sucralfate may decrease the absorption of these vitamins.

SIDE EFFECTS

NOT SERIOUS

NOT SERIOUS SIDE EFFECTS ARE RARE OR INFREQUENT. SEE WARNING, PAGE 27.

SERIOUS

- Unusual bruising, bleeding, or fatigue
- Rapid or irregular heartbeat
- Confusion, delirium, or hallucinations
- Shortness of breath
- Bronchospasm (tightness in the chest)
- Vomiting
- Vomit the consistency of coffee grounds
- Mouth ulcers
- Numbness or tingling in the fingers or toes
- Jaundice
- Severe abdominal pain accompanied by vomiting or fever (inflammation of the pancreas)
- Black, tarry stools (internal bleeding)
- Combined weakness, fever, and sore throat (bone marrow depression)

CONTACT YOUR DOCTOR IMMEDIATELY.

ATTAPULGITE

VITAL STATISTICS

DRUG CLASS
Antidiarrheal Drugs

BRAND NAME
Kaopectate

OTHER DRUGS IN THIS CLASS
bismuth subsalicylate, loperamide

GENERAL DESCRIPTION
Attapulgite is taken after each loose bowel movement to treat acute diarrhea that is mild to moderate. For chronic diarrhea, attapulgite should be used only for temporary relief of symptoms until the cause can be determined.

PRECAUTIONS

SPECIAL INFORMATION
- Since attapulgite is not absorbed into the body, it should not cause problems during pregnancy or breast-feeding.
- Diarrhea can cause excessive fluid loss. Call your doctor as soon as possible if you have any signs of dehydration, including decreased urination, lightheadedness and dizziness, wrinkled skin, dryness of mouth, or increased thirst.
- When you use antidiarrheal drugs, it is vitally important that you replace lost fluids by drinking large quantities of water and other clear liquids (such as decaffeinated colas and tea, ginger ale, and broth). Eat only gelatin for the first 24 hours. The next day you may eat bland foods, such as bread, crackers, cooked cereals, and applesauce. Other beverages and foods may make the condition worse.

- Do not use antidiarrheals if you have a fever or if your stool contains blood or mucus: These are symptoms of dysentery, an infection of the lower intestinal tract. Call your doctor.
- Antidiarrheal drugs have different functions. Some combat the symptoms of diarrhea; others are directed against the cause. A number of antidiarrheal drugs are available only by prescription. If over-the-counter medications do not help, see your doctor.

POSSIBLE INTERACTIONS
The presence of attapulgite in your body might prevent the absorption of other medications. Avoid taking other medications within two to three hours of taking attapulgite.

TARGET AILMENTS

Mild-to-moderate acute diarrhea

Traveler's diarrhea

SIDE EFFECTS

WHEN USED AT THE RECOMMENDED DOSAGE FOR NO MORE THAN TWO DAYS, ATTAPULGITE AND OTHER ANTIDIARRHEAL DRUGS RARELY CAUSE SIDE EFFECTS. BUT IF THE DIARRHEA DOES NOT DECREASE WITHIN ONE OR TWO DAYS, CHECK WITH YOUR DOCTOR.

NOT SERIOUS
- Mild constipation

CHECK WITH YOUR DOCTOR IF THE CONSTIPATION CONTINUES OR IF YOU DEVELOP A FEVER.

BACITRACIN

VITAL STATISTICS

DRUG CLASS
Antibiotics [Topical Antibiotics]

BRAND NAME
Neosporin

OTHER DRUGS IN THIS SUBCLASS
Rx: chlorhexidine (for gums); mupirocin (for skin); combination of neomycin, polymyxin B, and hydrocortisone (antibiotic-corticosteroid for ears)
OTC: neomycin, polymyxin B

GENERAL DESCRIPTION
Bacitracin is available by itself and in combination with neomycin and polymyxin B as an over-the-counter topical antibiotic. This combination and other over-the-counter topical antibiotics are available in an ointment base that helps close and soothe wounds. In general, though, the primary purpose of such OTC drugs is to guard against possible infections in minor cuts, scrapes, and burns. Once a skin infection is under way, your doctor may prescribe a stronger medication.

PRECAUTIONS

SPECIAL INFORMATION
- Check with your doctor if you notice no improvement after using these medications for two or three days.
- The use of topical antibiotics increases the risk of kidney damage or hearing loss in people with impaired kidney function who are already taking nephrotoxic medicines.
- If you are pregnant or nursing, check with your doctor before using.

POSSIBLE INTERACTIONS
None expected.

TARGET AILMENTS
Minor cuts, scrapes, and burns

SIDE EFFECTS

NOT SERIOUS
- Itching, stinging, rash, redness, or swelling at the application site

CALL YOUR DOCTOR IF THESE SYMPTOMS PERSIST OR ARE BOTHERSOME.

BEE POLLEN

VITAL STATISTICS

GENERAL DESCRIPTION

The nutritional components of bee pollen, which is extracted by professional methods from hives, include vitamin C, B-complex vitamins, amino acids, carotene, calcium, copper, iron, magnesium, and potassium. Although its benefits have not been scientifically proved, bee pollen is said to boost physical energy and endurance, and athletes sometimes take it to improve their performance. It may also relieve stress, fatigue, and depression, and aid in weight-loss efforts. Although it is reputed to help with respiratory allergies, it should not be taken by anyone allergic to bee stings.

Bee pollen has a germ-killing effect, and ailments for which it may be beneficial include bowel problems, cancer, heart ailments, and arthritis, although no scientific studies support such claims. It thus remains somewhat controversial as a health promoter.

NATURAL SOURCES

Flowering plants

PREPARATIONS

Available in capsules and by injection.

PRECAUTIONS

☠ WARNING

Do not use bee pollen if you are allergic to bee stings. Do not use if you have gout or kidney disease. Do not give to children under the age of two.

Do not use if you are pregnant or planning a pregnancy. If you are breast-feeding, do not use except under the advice of your healthcare practitioner.

SPECIAL INFORMATION

- Standard dosages and possible side effects of bee pollen have not been determined thoroughly. Begin with small amounts and discontinue if any allergic reactions occur.
- Those who are allergic to airborne pollen may wish to avoid taking bee pollen as a supplement, although the effects are not necessarily the same.
- Some commercial flower-pollen preparations do not contain pollen collected from bees. They are similar to bee pollen and may provide health benefits, although these too have yet to be proved.

TARGET AILMENTS

See General Description (left).

SIDE EFFECTS

NOT SERIOUS

- Rash
- Itching
- Pain at injection site
- Swelling

  DISCONTINUE USE AND CALL YOUR DOCTOR.

SERIOUS

- Anaphylactic shock (a severe allergic reaction indicated by extreme itching, swelling, loss of breath, lowered blood pressure, and loss of consciousness)

STAY WITH THE VICTIM, ADMINISTER CPR, AND HAVE SOMEONE CALL 911 OR YOUR EMERGENCY NUMBER.

BENZOCAINE

VITAL STATISTICS

DRUG CLASS
Anesthetics

BRAND NAMES
Anbesol, Orajel

OTHER DRUGS IN THIS CLASS
dyclonine, pramoxine

GENERAL DESCRIPTION
Benzocaine is an over-the-counter local anesthetic (derived from the same source as the sunscreen preparation PABA) that is frequently used to relieve pain and discomfort in the mouth and on the skin or mucous membranes. The drug works by deadening nerve endings so that they do not transmit pain messages to the brain. Most side effects associated with local anesthetics are caused by excessive applications or by individual sensitivity to the anesthetic. Benzocaine is more likely to cause sensitivity reactions than most other anesthetics.

PRECAUTIONS

SPECIAL INFORMATION
- Benzocaine should not be used on areas where irritation, infection, or bleeding is present unless your doctor directs you to do so. Benzocaine can cause excess irritation or become absorbed into the bloodstream, leading to overdose symptoms.
- Do not use benzocaine if you are sensitive or allergic to PABA, since the two are chemically similar.

POSSIBLE INTERACTIONS
None expected.

TARGET AILMENTS

Canker sores

Mouth or gum injury

Toothache

Pain from dental procedures or appliances

Pain associated with other minor skin and mouth problems

SIDE EFFECTS

SERIOUS
- Allergic reactions such as skin rash, hives, redness, and itching at the site of application
- Large hivelike swellings on the skin or in the mouth or throat
- Burning, stinging, and swelling not present before application

THESE SYMPTOMS ARE RARE. CALL YOUR DOCTOR TO DETERMINE WHETHER YOU USED TOO MUCH MEDICATION OR ARE SENSITIVE TO BENZOCAINE.

- Overdose symptoms including dizziness, headache, tiredness, blurred vision, irregular heartbeat, or ringing in the ears

CALL YOUR DOCTOR IMMEDIATELY.

BIOTIN

VITAL STATISTICS

OTHER NAMES
vitamin B$_7$, vitamin H

GENERAL DESCRIPTION
Along with other B vitamins, biotin helps convert food to energy and is required for the synthesis of carbohydrates, proteins, and fatty acids. Biotin is especially important for healthy hair, skin, and nails.
Biotin deficiency is rare, and supplements are unnecessary.

EMDR
30 mcg to 100 mcg

NATURAL SOURCES
Among the types of food that are good dietary sources of biotin are cheese, kidneys, salmon, soybeans, sunflower seeds, nuts, broccoli, and sweet potatoes.

PRECAUTIONS

SPECIAL INFORMATION
- Because breast milk contains little biotin, infants who are breast-fed can suffer biotin deficiency, although this is uncommon.
- Signs of biotin deficiency include dry, grayish skin; hair loss; nausea; vomiting; muscle pain; loss of appetite; a pale, smooth tongue; and fatigue.
- People can become biotin deficient through long-term use of antibiotics or by regularly eating raw egg whites, which contain avidin, a protein that blocks the body's absorption of biotin. Research has not revealed a toxic level for biotin.

TARGET AILMENTS

Immune problems

Skin problems

SIDE EFFECTS
NONE EXPECTED

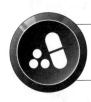

BISMUTH SUBSALICYLATE

VITAL STATISTICS

DRUG CLASS
Antidiarrheal Drugs

BRAND NAME
Pepto-Bismol

OTHER DRUGS IN THIS CLASS
attapulgite, loperamide

GENERAL DESCRIPTION
Bismuth subsalicylate is used to treat diarrhea. Because it appears to inhibit intestinal secretions, it is also effective in preventing symptoms of traveler's (infectious) diarrhea and can be taken regularly during the first two weeks of travel. This drug is also used to treat symptoms of gastric distress or upset stomach, including heartburn, acid indigestion, and nausea; it is also used in combination with antibiotics to treat duodenal ulcers.

PRECAUTIONS

SPECIAL INFORMATION
- Advise your healthcare professional if you have had allergic reactions to other salicylates, including aspirin.
- Do not give this drug to children without the approval of a doctor.
- If taken in higher doses and for longer periods to prevent traveler's diarrhea, bismuth subsalicylate may intensify some of the symptoms of dysentery, gout, kidney disease, stomach ulcers, and hemophilia and other bleeding problems. If you have any of these conditions, consult your doctor first before taking the drug.

- Bismuth subsalicylate may have an effect on some laboratory tests. Be sure to tell the healthcare practitioner performing the test that you are taking the medication.

POSSIBLE INTERACTIONS
Antidiabetic drugs (oral): may reduce blood sugar levels.
Tetracycline: reduced tetracycline absorption.

TARGET AILMENTS

Diarrhea, especially traveler's (infectious) diarrhea

Upset stomach

Heartburn; acid indigestion; nausea

SIDE EFFECTS

WHEN USED AT THE RECOMMENDED DOSAGE FOR NO MORE THAN TWO DAYS, THIS DRUG RARELY CAUSES SIDE EFFECTS. BUT IF THE DIARRHEA DOES NOT SUBSIDE WITHIN ONE OR TWO DAYS, CHECK WITH YOUR DOCTOR.

NOT SERIOUS
- Mild constipation
- Grayish black stools and darkened tongue

THESE EFFECTS ARE HARMLESS, BUT CHECK WITH YOUR DOCTOR IF THE CONSTIPATION CONTINUES OR YOU DEVELOP A FEVER.

BLUE-GREEN ALGAE

VITAL STATISTICS

OTHER NAME
spirulina

GENERAL DESCRIPTION
Blue-green algae is widely promoted as a tonic supplement that can be taken regularly for general health. It contains iron and vitamin B_{12} as well as amino acids; its nutritive value is sometimes compared to that of the soybean. Blue-green algae is said to have a blood-cleansing, rejuvenating effect, and it is touted as a low-fat, high-protein supplement that can increase energy levels, enhance mental alertness, and help curb the appetite. The broad claims associated with blue-green algae include its ability to boost the immune system, treat AIDS, and control Alzheimer's disease and diabetes mellitus.

Although anecdotal accounts suggest that some people benefit from these supplements, no scientific studies support claims of its curative powers. Some nutritionists describe blue-green algae as mere "pond scum" that has no medicinal value, contains only minuscule amounts of protein, and tastes horrible. The most widely known commercial product is spirulina, a type of blue-green algae packaged in Mexico, Japan, Thailand, and California.

NATURAL SOURCES
alkaline ponds and lakes

PREPARATIONS
Available as a tablet or a capsule.

PRECAUTIONS

☠ WARNING
Do not take blue-green algae if you are pregnant, planning a pregnancy, or breast-feeding. Do not give to children under the age of two.

SPECIAL INFORMATION
- Thoroughly research the product you intend to buy. Some preparations contain toxins, and others may be labeled as containing spirulina when in fact they do not.
- No standard recommended dosage has been determined for blue-green algae. Consult your doctor for dosages.

POSSIBLE INTERACTIONS
None expected for spirulina, considered the safest type of blue-green algae.

TARGET AILMENTS
Obesity

Fatigue

SIDE EFFECTS

SERIOUS
- Nausea
- Vomiting
- Diarrhea

DISCONTINUE USE AND CONSULT YOUR DOCTOR.

BREWER'S YEAST

VITAL STATISTICS

OTHER NAME
nutritional yeast

GENERAL DESCRIPTION
Brewer's yeast, a nonleavening yeast grown from hops, is valued as a source of protein, phosphorus, chromium, and B vitamins (it does not contain B_{12}, however). In small doses, the supplement is considered safe for growing children and older adults. Sold as a powder or in tablets or flakes, it is easily incorporated into cooked dishes, and it can be added to beverages or taken between meals for a quick energy boost.

The supplement contains trace amounts of the mineral chromium, which helps regulate blood sugar in diabetics. One to two teaspoons of brewer's yeast a day may help aid in weight loss by reducing cravings for sweets. The supplement is often recommended for skin problems such as eczema, and as a bulking agent it can be an effective remedy for constipation. Brewer's yeast is said to have an immune-building effect, and, although its effectiveness has not been determined, some practitioners recommend it to help treat diabetes, high cholesterol, and cancer.

NATURAL SOURCES
hops

PREPARATIONS
Available as a powder, tablets, or flakes.

PRECAUTIONS

☠ WARNING
Do not use brewer's yeast if you have candidiasis.

SPECIAL INFORMATION
No standard recommended dosage has been determined for brewer's yeast. Consult your doctor for dosages.

POSSIBLE INTERACTIONS
Do not combine brewer's yeast with other medications or herbal therapies except under the advice of your doctor.

TARGET AILMENTS

Eczema

Nervousness

Fatigue

Heart problems

Diabetes

Constipation

SIDE EFFECTS

NOT SERIOUS
- Headache
- Upset stomach; nausea
- Diarrhea

DISCONTINUE USE AND CALL YOUR DOCTOR.

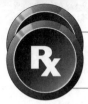

BRONCHODILATORS

VITAL STATISTICS

GENERIC NAMES
Rx: albuterol, epinephrine, ipratropium, salmeterol, terbutaline, theophylline
OTC: ephedrine, epinephrine, theophylline

GENERAL DESCRIPTION
Bronchodilators relax the muscles surrounding the bronchial tubes in the lungs by stimulating or inhibiting certain body chemicals. This relieves spasm and improves lung capacity, thereby alleviating the symptoms of bronchial asthma and bronchitis.

Theophylline (found naturally in commercial tea and related to the caffeine found in coffee) acts mainly on the muscles of the respiratory tract. Other bronchodilators act on the sinuses and upper respiratory tract as well. All of these drugs may act on the heart, arteries, and veins, especially if taken in large doses. For this reason, bronchodilators can affect blood pressure and heart function.

PRECAUTIONS

☠ WARNING
Your body can build up tolerance to bronchodilators used as inhalants, causing them to become less effective. If this happens, discontinue the drug and tell your doctor. Do not increase the dose, since this can lead to serious, perhaps fatal bronchial constriction.

SPECIAL INFORMATION
- These drugs (especially ephedrine and epinephrine) can cause adverse effects in individuals with high blood pressure, diabetes, heart disease, seizures, peptic ulcers, or thyroid or prostate problems. If you have any of these conditions do not use bronchodilators—even in their over-the-counter forms—without your doctor's permission.
- Women who are pregnant or breast-feeding should consult a doctor before using these drugs.

TARGET AILMENTS

Anaphylactic shock from severe allergic reactions

Acute bronchial asthma

Chronic, recurrent bronchial asthma

Bronchitis

Emphysema

Hay fever and cold symptoms (ephedrine)

Other chronic obstructive pulmonary diseases

Heart-rhythm problems and cardiac arrest (epinephrine)

Exercise-induced bronchospasm

BRONCHODILATORS

POSSIBLE INTERACTIONS

Alcohol: increased effect of theophylline, possibly causing theophylline toxicity.

Alpha and beta blockers: these drugs decrease the action of bronchodilators, especially ephedrine and epinephrine.

Blood pressure medicines, including diuretics: bronchodilators may decrease the actions of these medicines.

Caffeine and other central nervous system stimulants: increased nervousness and insomnia.

Diabetes medications, including insulin: decreased effectiveness of diabetes medications.

Heart medications (such as digoxin): heart-rhythm problems.

Levodopa: increased heart-rhythm problems. Your doctor may need to adjust your dosage.

Lithium: theophylline may decrease the effectiveness of lithium.

MAO inhibitors: possible effects on the heart or blood vessels.

Nitrates: decreased effectiveness of nitrates in relieving angina.

Other antiasthmatic drugs: do not combine these drugs unless your doctor directs you to do so or unless your prescription contains a combination. Using two bronchodilators may increase the side effects, especially on the heart.

Phenytoin: serious cardiovascular effects, such as heart-rhythm problems or very low blood pressure.

Thyroid medications: increased bronchodilator effect.

Tricyclic antidepressants and maprotiline: increased effects of bronchodilators on the cardiovascular system.

SIDE EFFECTS

NOT SERIOUS

- Mild nausea
- Mild weakness
- Insomnia
- Mild nervousness
- Restlessness

CALL YOUR DOCTOR IF THESE EFFECTS BECOME BOTHERSOME.

SERIOUS

- Change in blood pressure, change in heartbeat (irregular or pounding, for example)
- Trembling
- Breathing problems
- Weakness
- Anxiety; nervousness
- Dizziness; lightheadedness
- Muscle cramps
- Nausea or vomiting
- Chest pain or discomfort (rare)

LET YOUR DOCTOR KNOW RIGHT AWAY IF YOU EXPERIENCE THESE SIDE EFFECTS.

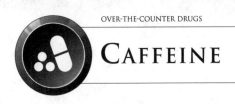

CAFFEINE

VITAL STATISTICS

BRAND NAMES
Vivarin; Anacin, Excedrin Extra-Strength
(combined with aspirin)

GENERAL DESCRIPTION
Caffeine, obtained from both natural and synthetic sources, has been used for centuries as a mild central nervous system stimulant. It works by stimulating all parts of the central nervous system, affecting the heart, lungs, other organs, and muscles. Caffeine also affects the blood vessels by temporarily increasing the heart's rate, contraction force, and output. While these effects usually produce no change in blood pressure for healthy individuals, you should avoid caffeine if you have high blood pressure.

Some over-the-counter analgesic drugs combine aspirin or acetaminophen with caffeine to enhance the painkilling effects of the analgesic.

Caffeine increases the production of stomach acids. Other effects include a slight diuretic action, a decrease in uterine contractions, and a temporary increase in blood sugar. Some people develop a tolerance to caffeine. When caffeine is used for a long period, abrupt discontinuation can produce withdrawal symptoms such as headache, irritability, dizziness, and unusual tiredness.

PRECAUTIONS

SPECIAL INFORMATION
- There has been some controversy regarding the use of caffeine by pregnant or nursing women. Although no proof of birth defects has been found, caffeine does cross the placenta, and small amounts also pass into breast milk. Caffeine can cause hyperactivity and insomnia in infants. For this reason, pregnant and nursing women should use caution and limit their intake of caffeine.
- Caffeine's effects on children have not been studied.

POSSIBLE INTERACTIONS
There is some evidence of interactions between caffeine and the following drugs: barbiturates, ulcer medications, antacids and supplements containing calcium, erythromycin, troleandomycin, and oral contraceptives. However, the effects of caffeine on the metabolizing of these medications are not well characterized in research studies and may not be clinically signficant.

TARGET AILMENTS
Fatigue

Pain (when used as an adjunctive, or additive, treatment in combination with analgesics such as aspirin)

Migraine and other vascular headaches (used with ergot preparations)

Beta blockers: combining these drugs may decrease the action of both.

Bronchodilators: taking caffeine with these may increase stimulation and other side effects.

Disulfiram (for alcohol dependency): may decrease the elimination of caffeine, thus intensifying its effects.

Grapefruit juice: possible increased caffeine effect.

Iron supplements: decreased iron absorption.

Lithium: may increase lithium elimination, decreasing lithium's effectiveness.

MAO inhibitors: combining with large amounts of caffeine may produce heart arrhythmias or severe hypertension.

Other central nervous system stimulants (amphetamines, pseudoephedrine): may add to stimulation and other adverse effects.

Other sources of caffeine or theobromines (related to caffeine) such as tea, coffee, chocolate: may produce an additive effect, making side effects more likely.

SIDE EFFECTS

NOT SERIOUS

- Mild stimulation of the central nervous system (jitters)
- Mild digestive upset or nausea
- Insomnia

CALL YOUR DOCTOR IF THESE SYMPTOMS BECOME BOTHERSOME.

SERIOUS

- Dizziness, increased heart rate, nervousness or tremors
- Digestive upsets such as nausea, vomiting, diarrhea

LET YOUR DOCTOR KNOW IF YOU HAVE THESE EFFECTS. YOU MAY HAVE TAKEN TOO MUCH CAFFEINE. OVERDOSE SYMPTOMS INCLUDE THOSE ABOVE PLUS HEADACHE, VISION DISTURBANCES SUCH AS SEEING FLASHES OR LIGHTS, DELIRIUM, FEVER, INCREASED SENSITIVITY TO PAIN, RINGING IN EARS.

CALCIUM

VITAL STATISTICS

GENERAL DESCRIPTION

Calcium, the most abundant mineral in the body, is essential for the growth and maintenance of bones and teeth. It enables muscles, including your heart, to contract; it is necessary for normal blood clotting, proper nerve-impulse transmission, and connective-tissue maintenance. It helps keep blood pressure normal and may reduce the risk of heart disease; taken with vitamin D, it may help lessen the risk of colorectal cancer. (*Caution:* Because vitamin D is toxic in high doses, this combination should be taken only if prescribed by a doctor.) It helps prevent rickets in children and osteoporosis in adults.

Different people need calcium in varying amounts. Supplemental calcium is available in many forms; the form that is best absorbed by the body is calcium citrate-malate.

RDA

Adults: 800 mg
Pregnant women and young adults: 1,200 mg

NATURAL SOURCES

Good sources of calcium include dairy products, dark green leafy vegetables, sardines, salmon, soy, and almonds.

PRECAUTIONS

☠ WARNING

Too much calcium can lead to constipation and to calcium deposits in soft tissue, causing damage to the heart, liver, or kidneys.

SPECIAL INFORMATION

- A sedentary lifestyle and consuming too much alcohol, dietary fiber, and fat can interfere with calcium absorption; too much protein and caffeine results in calcium being excreted in urine.
- For calcium to be properly absorbed, the body must have sufficient levels of vitamin D and of hydrochloric acid in the stomach, and a balance of other minerals, including magnesium and phosphorus.

TARGET AILMENTS

Osteoporosis in adults

Rickets in children

Colorectal cancer (when taken with vitamin D and if prescribed by a doctor)

Calcium helps regulate blood pressure and may reduce the risk of heart disease

SIDE EFFECTS
NONE EXPECTED

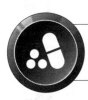

CALCIUM CARBONATE

VITAL STATISTICS

DRUG CLASS
Antacids

BRAND NAMES
Rolaids, Tums

OTHER DRUGS IN THIS CLASS
aluminum hydroxide, magnesium carbonate, magnesium hydroxide, sodium bicarbonate and citric acid

GENERAL DESCRIPTION
Calcium carbonate is a calcium-containing antacid drug that relieves symptoms of upset and sour stomach, heartburn, acid indigestion, and ulcers. Calcium carbonate is most effective when taken on an empty stomach. This medication is also used to help prevent calcium-deficiency diseases such as osteoporosis. See Antacids for more information, including possible drug interactions.

PRECAUTIONS

SPECIAL INFORMATION
- Except under special circumstances determined by your doctor, antacids should not be used if you have impaired renal function or high levels of calcium in your blood, a condition known as hypercalcemia.
- Notify your doctor if you develop symptoms such as black, tarry stools or vomit the consistency of coffee grounds. These are indications of bleeding in the stomach or intestines.
- Calcium carbonate can cause milk-alkali syndrome, which is characterized by headaches, nausea, irritability, and weakness. In time, milk-alkali syndrome can lead to kidney disease or kidney failure.

TARGET AILMENTS

Upset stomach; heartburn; acid indigestion; sour stomach

Ulcers

Calcium deficiency

SIDE EFFECTS

NOT SERIOUS
- Mild constipation
- Laxative effect or diarrhea
- Chalky taste in the mouth
- Stomach cramps; nausea
- Belching
- Flatulence
- White specks in the stool

CALL YOUR DOCTOR IF THESE PROBLEMS PERSIST.

SERIOUS
- Swelling of the wrist, foot, or lower leg
- Bone pain
- Severe constipation
- Dizziness
- Mood changes
- Muscle pain, weakness, or twitching
- Slow breathing
- Irregular heartbeat
- Fatigue
- Pain upon urinating or frequent need to urinate
- Change in appetite

CONTACT YOUR DOCTOR IMMEDIATELY.

CALCIUM POLYCARBOPHIL

VITAL STATISTICS

DRUG CLASS
Laxatives

BRAND NAME
FiberCon

OTHER DRUGS IN THIS CLASS
methylcellulose, psyllium hydrophilic mucilloid

GENERAL DESCRIPTION
Calcium polycarbophil is a bulk-forming laxative used for the temporary relief of both constipation and diarrhea, and to prevent straining during bowel movements. Bulk-forming laxatives, considered the safest and therefore the first choice in treating constipation, work by absorbing water and expanding, thus increasing the moisture content of the stool to make passage easier. They may also be especially beneficial to people on low-fiber diets and to those with irritable bowel syndrome (spastic colon), diverticulitis, or hemorrhoids. See Laxatives for more information, including possible drug interactions.

PRECAUTIONS

SPECIAL INFORMATION
- When taking this laxative, be sure to drink plenty of water or other fluid to avoid obstruction of the throat and esophagus. Taking this medication without enough liquid may cause choking.
- You may not experience the effects of this laxative for 12 to 72 hours after taking it.
- Bulk-forming laxatives are best for geriatric patients with poorly functioning colons.

- If you have difficulty swallowing, do not take bulk-forming laxatives, which can cause an esophageal obstruction.
- Call your doctor if this drug fails to have the desired effect after one week of use.

POSSIBLE INTERACTIONS
Laxatives that may contain danthron, mineral oil, or phenolphthalein: increased absorption of these substances, increasing the possibility of toxic effects.
Oral anticoagulants, digitalis, salicylate, tetracycline: these drugs may be less effective when taken concurrently with bulk-forming laxatives. After taking any of these drugs, wait two hours before taking a laxative.

TARGET AILMENTS

Constipation

Diarrhea

Irritable bowel syndrome (spastic colon)

Straining during bowel movements following rectal surgery or heart attacks, or when hemorrhoids are present

SIDE EFFECTS

NOT SERIOUS
- Harmless urine discoloration
- Skin rash

CHAMOMILE

LATIN NAME
Matricaria recutita

VITAL STATISTICS

GENERAL DESCRIPTION
Of the three types of chamomile plant, the most popular and thoroughly studied is German chamomile, used medicinally around the world for thousands of years. Modern herbalists have identified elements in the oil of the chamomile flower that appear to calm the central nervous system, relax the digestive tract, and speed the healing process.

PREPARATIONS
Over the counter:
Available as prepared tea, tincture, essential oil, and dried or fresh flowers.

At home:
TEA: Pour 8 oz boiling water over 2 tsp chamomile flowers and steep for 10 minutes. Drink 1 cup three or four times daily, or dilute and use as an eye compress.
EYE COMPRESS: Strain the tea through a coffee filter and dilute with an equal amount of water. Always use fresh tea (less than 24 hours old) and refrigerate unused portions. (Bring the dilute tea to room temperature before using it.) To make the compress, pour the liquid on a cloth and apply to the closed eye. Discontinue if your eye becomes irritated.
FOMENTATION: Apply three or four times daily to sore muscles; sore, swollen joints; varicose veins; and burns and skin wounds.
HERBAL BATH: Run bathwater over 2 or 3 oz chamomile flowers tied in cloth, or add no more than 2 drops essential oil of chamomile to bathwater.
Consult a practitioner for the dosage appropriate for you and the specific ailment.

PRECAUTIONS

SPECIAL INFORMATION
Allergies to chamomile are rare. However, anyone allergic to other plants in the daisy family (chrysanthemum, ragweed, and aster, for example) should be alert to possible allergic reactions to chamomile, ranging from contact dermatitis to life-threatening anaphylaxis (itching, rash, and difficulty in breathing).

POSSIBLE INTERACTIONS
Combining chamomile with other herbs may necessitate a lower dosage.

TARGET AILMENTS

Take internally for:

Stomach cramps, gas, nervous stomach, indigestion, ulcers, colic; menstrual cramps; insomnia; anxiety

Apply externally for:

Joint swelling and pain; skin inflammation; sunburn; cuts and scrapes; teething pain; varicose veins; hemorrhoids; sore or inflamed eyes

Use as a gargle for:

Gingivitis; sore throat

SIDE EFFECTS
NONE EXPECTED

CHARCOAL, ACTIVATED

VITAL STATISTICS

BRAND NAMES
Charcocaps, Actidose-Aqua, Charcodote, Liquid-Antidose, Charcosalanti Dote

DAILY DOSAGE
For diarrhea or gas pain, 2 capsules three or four times a day
For gout, 1 tsp three times a day

GENERAL DESCRIPTION
Activated charcoal, a type of chemically treated carbon used in medicine, has little in common with the charcoal used on the grill. Activated charcoal takes the form of tiny particles suspended in water and is often used by doctors to cleanse the intestinal tract of toxic substances. It is sometimes given as an antidote for poisoning or for overdose of such medications as aspirin and acetaminophen.

Introduced into the body, activated charcoal attracts and collects toxins, then carries them out through the stool. Because it does not enter the bloodstream, charcoal is generally considered safe, and overdose is unlikely.

PREPARATIONS
Available in capsules, powder, or suspension.

PRECAUTIONS

☠ WARNING
Charcoal can interfere with the body's absorption of other drugs, particularly heart medications. Take activated charcoal at least two hours before or after taking other medications or vitamin supplements.

SPECIAL INFORMATION
- Contact a doctor in the case of poisoning. Do not try to treat the condition yourself.
- Heat and moisture can inhibit the action of charcoal. Store in a cool, dry place away from children.
- Women who are pregnant or breast-feeding should consult a doctor before using activated charcoal supplements.
- Although overdose is unlikely, if extreme amounts of charcoal are ingested, you should notify a doctor, emergency room, or poison control center right away.

TARGET AILMENTS

Diarrhea

Gout

Gas and gas pains

Poisoning and drug overdose

Hangover

Hiccups

SIDE EFFECTS

NOT SERIOUS
- Blackened stool; constipation; diarrhea; vomiting (if taken in large doses)

CHONDROITIN SULFATE

VITAL STATISTICS

GENERAL DESCRIPTION
Chondroitin sulfate is a complex carbohydrate that is produced naturally in the bodies of all mammals, including humans, and in parts of oysters and mussels. Most people have no need for additional amounts of the substance. But some, including individuals with weak bones or joints, heart problems, or arthritis, may benefit from supplements because chondroitin sulfate is thought to be an effective blood thinner and cell rejuvenator. A number of researchers think chondroitin sulfate can reduce the risk of blood clots and may help strengthen artery walls, bones, and joints. Some evidence suggests that chondroitin sulfate has antiviral properties as well.

A variety of claims have been made about chondroitin sulfate; it has been hailed as an effective antiaging drug, for example, and even as a mild aphrodisiac. So far, however, there is little scientific evidence that the substance has any real therapeutic effect.

NATURAL SOURCES
mussels, oysters, meat from mammals

PREPARATIONS
Chondroitin sulfate is available in capsule form at many health food stores.

PRECAUTIONS

☠ WARNING
Do not take chondroitin sulfate if you are pregnant, planning a pregnancy, or breast-feeding.

If you are taking anticoagulant drugs or have a blood-clotting disorder, consult your doctor before taking chondroitin sulfate.

Do not give this supplement to children under two years of age except upon the advice of a doctor.

SPECIAL INFORMATION
No standard recommended dosage has been determined for chondroitin sulfate. Consult your doctor for dosages.

POSSIBLE INTERACTIONS
Taking chondroitin sulfate may interfere with the action of prescription and nonprescription drugs, other supplements, or herbal therapies. Consult your doctor for guidance.

TARGET AILMENTS

Joint problems; weak cartilage; headache

Respiratory ailments; allergies

Arthritis; bursitis

SIDE EFFECTS
NONE EXPECTED

CHROMIUM

VITAL STATISTICS

GENERAL DESCRIPTION

As a component of a natural substance called glucose tolerance factor, chromium works with insulin to regulate the body's use of sugar and is essential to fatty-acid metabolism. Its contribution to metabolism makes chromium a helpful supplement in weight-loss programs.

Supplemental chromium may be used to treat some cases of adult-onset diabetes, to reduce insulin requirements of some diabetic children, and to relieve symptoms of hypoglycemia.

Inadequate chromium can result in alcohol intolerance, cause variable, inconsistent blood sugar levels, and possibly induce diabetes-like symptoms such as tingling in the extremities and reduced muscle coordination, or hypoglycemic symptoms such as fatigue and dizziness.

In addition, because chromium lowers cholesterol and triglyceride levels in both diabetic and nondiabetic subjects, deficiencies may result in an increased risk of atherosclerosis or cardiovascular disease.

EMDR

Adults: 50 mcg to 200 mcg

NATURAL SOURCES

Trace amounts of chromium are found in many foods, including brewer's yeast, liver, lean meats, poultry, molasses, whole grains, eggs, and cheese.

PRECAUTIONS

☠ WARNING

Taken regularly in supplements greater than 1,000 mcg, chromium inhibits insulin's activity and can be toxic to the liver and kidneys.

SPECIAL INFORMATION

Chromium is not absorbed well, so the body uses only a small portion of what is taken in through diet. Most people do not get enough dietary chromium, and some may benefit from a multinutrient supplement, such as chromium citrate or chromium picolinate. Nevertheless, care should be taken to avoid supplementing beyond the EMDR.

TARGET AILMENTS

Diabetes

Heart disease

Hypoglycemia

Alcoholism

SIDE EFFECTS

NONE EXPECTED

CIMETIDINE

DRUG CLASS
Antiulcer Drugs [Histamine H_2 Blockers]

BRAND NAMES
Rx: Tagamet
OTC: Tagamet HB

OTHER DRUGS IN THIS CLASS
lansoprazole, omeprazole, sucralfate
Histamine H_2 blockers: famotidine, nizatidine, ranitidine

GENERAL DESCRIPTION
Cimetidine is used both to treat and to prevent ulcers of the stomach and duodenum (upper intestine). It is also prescribed for other conditions characterized by an overproduction of stomach acid, such as Zollinger-Ellison syndrome and gastroesophageal reflux (in which stomach acid flows backward into the esophagus). In some cases, cimetidine is used to help stop upper gastrointestinal bleeding.

In the over-the-counter form, cimetidine is used not for ulcers but to relieve acid indigestion and heartburn. Although the OTC version is a lower dose of cimetidine than the prescription form, essentially the same interactions apply, though the side effects are milder.

Like other histamine H_2 blockers, cimetidine works by blocking the stomach's response to the chemical compound histamine, thereby reducing the secretion of the digestive juice hydrochloric acid. For more information on side effects and possible drug interactions, see Antiulcer Drugs.

SPECIAL INFORMATION
- Inform your doctor if you have a history of arthritis, kidney or liver disease, organic brain syndrome, asthma, or low sperm count.
- Avoid this drug if you are pregnant or nursing.
- Cimetidine may affect the results of some medical tests, including blood cholesterol levels, liver function tests, and sperm counts. Inform the person giving you the test that you are taking this medication.
- This drug may inhibit your body's ability to absorb vitamin B_{12}. Talk to your doctor about B_{12} supplements.

TARGET AILMENTS
Duodenal ulcer

Gastric ulcer

Upper gastrointestinal bleeding associated with gastric ulcer or duodenal ulcer, or with gastritis

Zollinger-Ellison syndrome

Multiple endocrine neoplasia

Other conditions characterized by an overproduction of stomach acid

Gastroesophageal reflux

Acid indigestion and heartburn (OTC)

CONTINUED

CIMETIDINE

POSSIBLE INTERACTIONS

This drug interacts with many prescription and over-the-counter medications, some of which are listed here. Make sure you inform your doctor of any other drugs you may be taking.

Alcohol: cimetidine may interfere with the elimination of alcohol from the body, prolonging alcohol's intoxicating effects.

Antacids: blocked absorption of cimetidine; space dosages of cimetidine and antacids at least an hour apart.

Anticoagulants (such as warfarin), oral anti-diabetic drugs, benzodiazepines, calcium channel blockers (such as amlodipine and diltiazem), carbamazepine, cyclosporine, lidocaine, metoprolol, pentoxifylline, phenytoin, procainamide, propranolol, quinidine, theophylline, triamterene, tricyclic antidepressants: increased effects of these drugs, possibly leading to toxicity.

Carmustine: increased risk of blood disorders.

Enteric-coated tablets: changes in stomach acidity may cause these drugs to dissolve prematurely in the stomach; avoid taking enteric-coated medications with cimetidine.

Itraconazole, ketoconazole, tetracycline: decreased absorption of these drugs into the body.

Sucralfate: decreased absorption of cimetidine.

Tobacco (smoking): may block the beneficial effects of cimetidine.

SIDE EFFECTS

NOT SERIOUS

- Mild diarrhea
- Mild skin rash or hives
- Dizziness
- Headache
- Blurred vision
- Fatigue
- Muscle and joint pain

CONTACT YOUR DOCTOR IF THESE SYMPTOMS CONTINUE OR BECOME BOTHERSOME.

SERIOUS

- Confusion
- Nervousness
- Delirium and hallucinations
- Slowed or irregular heartbeat
- Abnormal bleeding or bruising
- Combined weakness, fever, and sore throat (signs of bone marrow depression)
- Hair loss
- Rash
- Enlarged or painful breasts (in women or men)
- Male impotence
- Jaundice

CALL YOUR DOCTOR IMMEDIATELY.

COENZYME Q10

VITAL STATISTICS

OTHER NAME
ubiquinone

DAILY DOSAGE
Usually 50 mg to 150 mg, though higher doses are sometimes used. Check with your doctor for the dosage that is appropriate for you.

GENERAL DESCRIPTION
An antioxidant involved in the production of energy in cells, coenzyme Q10 (CoQ10) is sometimes called ubiquinone, from the word ubiquitous, because it is found in cells throughout the body. Levels of CoQ10 decrease as a person ages, a fact that leads some nutritionists to speculate that supplementation might slow down the aging process. In Japan, CoQ10 is used extensively to reduce the risk of heart attack, lower blood pressure, treat congestive heart failure, and boost the immune system. Some research suggests that supplements are useful in treating angina and may help prevent heart damage after surgery.

PREPARATIONS
CoQ10 is sold in the United States as a dietary supplement in the form of capsules, tablets, and soft gelatin capsules.

Keep CoQ10 cool and dry and away from light, and don't allow it to freeze.

SIDE EFFECTS
NONE EXPECTED

PRECAUTIONS

☠ WARNING
Do not take CoQ10 supplements if you are pregnant or breast-feeding.

SPECIAL INFORMATION
- Check labels carefully; not all products offer CoQ10 in its purest form.
- If you have heart disease, consult your doctor before taking supplements.

TARGET AILMENTS

Allergies; asthma

Alzheimer's disease

Cancer

Candidiasis

Cardiovascular disease; congestive heart failure; cardiomyopathy; angina pectoris

Diabetes mellitus

Hypertension

Muscular dystrophy

Obesity

Periodontal disease

Respiratory disease

Schizophrenia

COPPER

VITAL STATISTICS

GENERAL DESCRIPTION

Copper is indispensable to human health. Its many functions include the following: helping to form hemoglobin in the blood; facilitating the absorption and use of iron so red blood cells can transport oxygen to tissues; assisting in the regulation of blood pressure and heart rate; strengthening blood vessels, bones, tendons, and nerves; promoting fertility; and ensuring normal skin and hair pigmentation. Some evidence suggests that copper helps prevent cardiovascular problems such as high blood pressure and heart arrhythmias and that it may help treat arthritis and scoliosis. Copper may also protect tissue from damage by free radicals, support the body's immune function, and contribute to preventing cancer.

Excess calcium and zinc will interfere with copper absorption, but a true copper deficiency is rare and tends to be limited to people either with certain inherited diseases that inhibit copper absorption, such as albinism, or with acquired malabsorption ailments, such as Crohn's disease and celiac disease. The deficiency may also occur in infants who are not breast-fed and in some premature babies. Symptoms of copper deficiency include brittle, discolored hair; skeletal defects; anemia; high blood pressure; heart arrhythmias; and infertility.

Some research suggests that high levels of copper and iron may play a role in hyperactivity and autism.

Common supplemental forms are copper aspartate, copper citrate, and copper picolinate.

EMDR
Adults: 1.5 mg to 3 mg

NATURAL SOURCES

Most adults get enough copper from a normal, varied diet. Seafood and organ meats are the richest sources; blackstrap molasses, nuts, seeds, green vegetables, black pepper, cocoa, and water passed through copper pipes also contain significant quantities.

PRECAUTIONS

☠ WARNING
Supplemental copper should be taken only on a doctor's advice.

SPECIAL INFORMATION
- Taking more than 10 mg of copper daily can bring on nausea, vomiting, muscle pain, and stomachaches.
- Women who are pregnant or are taking birth-control pills are susceptible to excess blood levels of copper.

TARGET AILMENTS

Cancer

Heart disease

Immune problems

SIDE EFFECTS
NONE EXPECTED

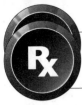

CORTICOSTEROIDS

GENERIC NAMES

Rx: beclomethasone, betamethasone, fluticasone, methylprednisolone, mometasone furoate, prednisone, triamcinolone
OTC: hydrocortisone

GENERAL DESCRIPTION

The term *corticosteroids* refers both to natural hormones produced by the adrenal glands and to synthetic versions of these hormones. Corticosteroids are powerful drugs, prescribed for a variety of conditions ranging in severity from skin rash to multiple sclerosis. Because they affect almost all parts of the body, these drugs must be used with caution.

Corticosteroid medications are available in topical creams, nasal inhalers and sprays, lung inhalers and sprays, and oral forms (tablets, syrup, and solutions).

PRECAUTIONS

SPECIAL INFORMATION

- Corticosteroid topical creams, as well as nasal and oral sprays or inhalers, may be absorbed into your system after prolonged use. Tell your doctor if you are taking any other medication, and watch for any significant side effects or drug interactions.
- Ask your doctor about the risks and benefits of corticosteroid treatment if you have or have had any of the following conditions: HIV infection or AIDS, heart disease, hypertension, ulcerative colitis, diabetes, diverticulitis, gastritis or peptic ulcers, recent chickenpox or measles, candidiasis or other fungal infections, glaucoma, herpes simplex, liver or kidney disease, myasthenia gravis, osteoporosis, anastomoses, lupus, tuberculosis, recent intestinal problems, or any infection, such as a cold or flu.
- Prolonged use of corticosteroids can cause birth defects. Pregnant and nursing women should avoid these drugs.
- Prolonged use of corticosteroids increases the risk of osteoporosis, cataracts, glaucoma, Cushing's syndrome (moon face), and diabetes. It can also reactivate tuberculosis.
- Check with your doctor before you stop using these drugs. It may be necessary to reduce the dosage gradually to avoid serious consequences.

POSSIBLE INTERACTIONS

Aminoglutethimide, antacids, barbiturates, phenytoin, and rifampin: decreased effectiveness of corticosteroids.
Diuretics: decreased effectiveness of both combined drugs.
Growth hormones, isoniazid, potassium supplements, and salicylates: corticosteroids may decrease the effectiveness of these drugs.
Oral anticoagulants: corticosteroids may increase or decrease the effectiveness of oral anticoagulants.
Vaccines (live virus, other immunizations): corticosteroids may make you more susceptible to the injected virus.

CONTINUED

CORTICOSTEROIDS

TARGET AILMENTS

Skin disorders, for symptomatic relief of rash, inflammation, itching; treatment of psoriasis, eczema, sunburn, and other skin diseases (hydrocortisone and mometasone furoate)

Nasal inflammations, including hay fever (allergic rhinitis) and nonallergic inflammation of the nasal passages (beclomethasone and triamcinolone)

Respiratory ailments such as severe asthma (beclomethasone and triamcinolone)

Rheumatic disorders (arthritis, bursitis, tendinitis); ulcerative colitis; Crohn's disease (prednisone)

Itchiness and inflammation associated with fungal infections such as athlete's foot, jock itch, and yeast infections (betamethasone, in combination with the antifungal drug clotrimazole)

SIDE EFFECTS

NOT SERIOUS

- Mild and transient skin rash, burning, irritation, dryness, redness, itchiness, or scaling (topical corticosteroids)
- Stomach upset; increased or decreased appetite; restlessness; dizziness; sleeplessness; change in skin color; unusual hair growth on face or body (other corticosteroids)

SERIOUS

- Eye pain
- Vision loss or blurred vision
- Stomach pain or burning sensation in the stomach
- Black, tarry stools
- Severe and lasting skin rash, hives, or burning, itching, or painful skin
- Blisters, acne, or other skin problems
- Nausea or vomiting
- High blood pressure
- Foot or leg swelling
- Rapid weight gain
- Fluid retention (edema)
- Unusual bruising
- Menstrual irregularities
- Prolonged sore throat, fever, cold, or other sign of infection

CONTACT YOUR DOCTOR IMMEDIATELY.

DECONGESTANTS

VITAL STATISTICS

GENERIC NAMES
Rx: phenylpropanolamine
OTC: oxymetazoline, phenylephrine, phenyl-propanolamine, pseudoephedrine

GENERAL DESCRIPTION
Available as sprays or pills in over-the-counter and prescription forms, decongestants relieve nasal and sinus congestion and headaches by constricting blood vessels in the nose and other parts of the respiratory system. Because the drugs affect certain receptors in the nervous system, high doses (doses above recommended amounts) may produce central nervous system side effects. Some of those medications used orally are chemically related to amphetamines and are banned for athletic use.

Decongestants come in both pill and spray forms; the form selected depends on the purpose to be achieved. Nasal sprays give the fastest results and are used for short-term treatment of nasal congestion. Use of these sprays for extended periods of time or at higher-than-recommended doses may result in nasal irritation or rebound congestion (nasal stuffiness, swelling, and redness without underlying illness).

In pill form, decongestants are used alone or in combination with other drugs to relieve the symptoms of colds, allergies, and other respiratory problems. Decongestant pills do not usually produce rebound congestion and therefore are useful for long-term treatment of nasal congestion. Decongestant pills can also be used to treat problems caused by pressure changes during air travel.

PRECAUTIONS

SPECIAL INFORMATION
- In rare cases, phenylpropanolamine has been associated with serious cardiovascular side effects, including severe high blood pressure and heart-rhythm problems, as well as psychotic problems, such as hallucinations and seizures. These effects are associated with high doses of phenylpropanolamine and may be more likely in individuals with similar preexisting problems, such as high blood pressure or neurological or psychiatric disease.
- Check with your doctor before taking any decongestants if you have cardiovascular disease (including angina, coronary artery disease, and hypertension), hyperthyroidism (overactive thyroid), diabetes, or glaucoma. Decongestants may exacerbate these conditions.

TARGET AILMENTS

Congestion of the nose and sinuses caused by allergy or upper respiratory infection

Congestion of Eustachian tubes, which join the ear with the nose and throat (pseudoephedrine)

Bronchial asthma (phenylpropanolamine)

Obesity (phenylpropanolamine, used as an appetite suppressant)

Urinary incontinence (phenylpropanolamine)

CONTINUED

DECONGESTANTS

POSSIBLE INTERACTIONS

Anticoagulant (blood-thinning) drugs: decreased anticoagulant effect.

Beta blockers: oral decongestants can lessen the effectiveness of beta blockers, causing hypertension.

Digitalis preparations: taking these drugs with oral decongestants may result in heart-rhythm problems.

High blood pressure drugs containing rauwolfia: decreased effectiveness of oral decongestants.

MAO inhibitors: increased stimulant action of oral decongestants, causing effects such as hypertension and heart-rhythm problems.

Stimulants (such as other decongestants, amphetamines, caffeine): increased stimulant effects, leading to excessive nervousness, insomnia, irregular heart rhythm, or seizures.

Tricyclic antidepressants (such as amitriptyline): increased action of oxymetazoline and phenylpropanolamine, making serious central nervous system side effects more likely.

SIDE EFFECTS

NOT SERIOUS

- Mild nervousness
- Mild restlessness
- Mild insomnia
- Dizziness
- Lightheadedness
- Nausea
- Dryness of mouth or nose
- Rebound congestion
- Sneezing; burning, stinging, or dryness of nose (spray and topical forms)

CALL YOUR DOCTOR IF THESE SYMPTOMS CONTINUE OR BECOME TROUBLESOME.

SERIOUS

- Severe headache
- Nervousness
- Restlessness
- Insomnia
- Pounding or irregular heartbeat
- High blood pressure

CONTACT YOUR DOCTOR IMMEDIATELY.

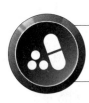

DEXTROMETHORPHAN

DRUG CLASS
Cough Suppressants

BRAND NAMES
Some types of Comtrex, Contac, and Thera-Flu; Benylin Adult Formula Cough Suppressant, Benylin DM Cough Syrup, Benylin Pediatric Cough Suppressant, Buckley's Mixture, Dextromethorphan Hydrobromide Cough Syrup, Dimetapp DM Elixir, DM Syrup, Drixoral Cough Liquid Caps, Hold DM 4 Hour Cough Relief, Iodrol, NyQuil, PediaCare (various forms), Pertussin CS, Robitussin Cough Calmers, Robitussin Pediatric Cough Suppressant, Robitussin Maximum Strength Cough Suppressant, Robitussin-CF, Robitussin-DM, St. Joseph Cough Suppressant for Children, Sucrets 4 Hour Cough Suppressant, Triaminic Nite Light, Triaminic Sore Throat Formula, Triaminic DM Syrup, Triaminicol Multi-Symptom Relief, Trocal, Tylenol Cold (adults and children), Vicks DayQuil Liquid or LiquiCaps, Vicks Pediatric Formula 44 Cough Medicine, Vicks Formula 44 Maximum Strength Cough Suppressant

GENERAL DESCRIPTION
Dextromethorphan is the main ingredient in a large number of widely available over-the-counter cough suppressants (antitussives) and common cold medications. The drug is used for the temporary relief of dry coughs caused by the common cold or flu. It should not be used for chronic coughs or for coughs that produce secretions.

Some cough suppressants act on the throat and bronchial passages to soothe irritation and relax the muscles. Others, including dextromethorphan, work in the brain to suppress the cough reflex. Like codeine, from which it is derived, dextromethorphan inhibits the cough reflex by acting directly on the cough center, located in the medulla of the brain. Unlike codeine, however, dextromethorphan is not a narcotic. When taken at the recommended dosages, it lacks analgesic and addictive properties and does not depress respiration.

CONTINUED

DEXTROMETHORPHAN

PRECAUTIONS

☠ *WARNING*

Overdose symptoms include confusion, hyperactivity, feeling of intoxication, lack of coordination, hallucinations, irritability, and severe nausea and vomiting. Seek immediate medical help.

SPECIAL INFORMATION

- Do not take dextromethorphan if you have had an allergic reaction to any medications containing this drug.
- Before taking dextromethorphan, consult your doctor if you have asthma or impaired liver function, or if your cough is producing mucus or phlegm.
- Use dextromethorphan only as instructed by your doctor or the directions on the label. Take it only as long as needed; some reports suggest that this drug may be habit forming if you use too much for too long.
- Check with your doctor if your cough persists for more than seven to 10 days or if it is accompanied by a skin rash, high fever, or continuing headache. These symptoms may indicate the presence of other medical problems.

POSSIBLE INTERACTIONS

Central nervous system depressants (anesthetics, antidepressants, antihistamines, anti-insomnia drugs, barbiturates, benzodiazepines, muscle relaxants, narcotics or prescription pain medicines, tranquilizers): increased sedative and depressant effects.

Monoamine oxidase (MAO) inhibitors: disorientation, psychotic behavior, coma.

TARGET AILMENTS

Dry, nonproductive, and temporary coughing

SIDE EFFECTS

NOT SERIOUS

- Mild drowsiness
- Mild dizziness
- Stomach pain
- Nausea
- Vomiting

CALL YOUR DOCTOR IF THESE SYMPTOMS PERSIST OR BECOME BOTHERSOME.

SERIOUS

ADVERSE EFFECTS AT THE RECOMMENDED NONPRESCRIPTION DOSAGES ARE MILD AND RARE. FOR OVERDOSE SYMPTOMS, SEE WARNING ABOVE, LEFT.

DGL

VITAL STATISTICS

OTHER NAME
deglycyrrhizinated licorice

DAILY DOSAGE
As directed.

GENERAL DESCRIPTION
When the substance glycyrrhizin is removed from the herb licorice root, a derivative known as deglycyrrhizinated licorice, or DGL, is formed. Glycyrrhizin, regarded as one of licorice root's most active ingredients, possesses many therapeutic properties for which licorice root is famous, such as anti-inflammatory, antiviral, and antidepressant properties. However, glycyrrhizin is also responsible for the harmful side effects associated with licorice, including high blood pressure, fluid retention, weakness, and irregular heart rate.

The derivative DGL causes none of the side effects associated with licorice root yet still offers healing benefits, especially in the treatment of peptic ulcers resulting from the overuse of aspirin, ibuprofen, caffeine, or alcohol. DGL helps increase mucous secretion, which helps protect the gastric lining, inhibiting the development of ulcers. DGL may be effective not only in treating existing ulcers but also in helping prevent injury to the stomach lining during long-term therapeutic use of aspirin or nonsteroidal anti-inflammatory drugs, or other medications that may tend to promote gastric ulcers.

PREPARATIONS
Available as a chewable tablet, liquid, or extract.

PRECAUTIONS

SPECIAL INFORMATION
- Since some ulcers need to be treated with antibiotics or other medications, consult your doctor if you think you have an ulcer.
- Do not give DGL supplements to children under two years of age except upon the advice of a doctor.
- If you have an existing medical condition or if you are pregnant, planning a pregnancy, or breast-feeding, consult your doctor before taking DGL supplements.

POSSIBLE INTERACTIONS
If you are taking any other supplements, prescription or nonprescription medications, or herbal therapies, consult your doctor before taking DGL supplements.

TARGET AILMENTS
Peptic ulcers

Mouth sores

SIDE EFFECTS
NONE EXPECTED

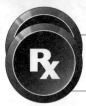

DIPHENHYDRAMINE

VITAL STATISTICS

DRUG CLASS
Antihistamines

BRAND NAMES
Rx: Benadryl
OTC: Benadryl, Excedrin PM, Tylenol Cold Night Time Medication Liquid, Tylenol PM, Unisom

OTHER DRUGS IN THIS CLASS
Rx: astemizole, cetirizine, fexofenadine, loratadine, promethazine, terfenadine
OTC: brompheniramine, chlorpheniramine, clemastine, dexbrompheniramine, doxylamine, triprolidine

GENERAL DESCRIPTION
Introduced in 1946, diphenhydramine was one of the first antihistamines. Its sedating and drying effects are more pronounced than those of the newer antihistamines. Diphenhydramine is used to treat symptoms of allergies, insomnia, chronic cough, vertigo, and mild Parkinson's disease. One form of diphenhydramine, a drug called dimenhydrinate, is used to treat motion sickness. See Antihistamines for additional information, including side effects.

PRECAUTIONS

SPECIAL INFORMATION
- Diphenhydramine causes drowsiness in varying degrees; avoid driving or operating machinery until you know how the drug affects you.
- Check with your doctor before using diphenhydramine if you have asthma, glaucoma, hyperthyroidism, high blood pressure, an enlarged prostate, a stomach ulcer, a bladder obstruction, or heart disease; this drug may exacerbate these conditions.
- Diphenhydramine is not recommended for pregnant and breast-feeding women. Consult your doctor and use only if clearly needed.

POSSIBLE INTERACTIONS
Alcohol: likely to increase the sedative effects of dipenhydramine; do not drink when you take these drugs.
Antianxiety drugs; barbiturates or other sedatives: do not take with antihistamines, as the combination may result in excessive sedation.
MAO inhibitors: can cause hypotension and dryness of the respiratory passages when taken with antihistamines. Do not combine these with antihistamines.

TARGET AILMENTS

Nasal and respiratory allergies (seasonal and nonseasonal), including hay fever

Common cold (used in combination with other drugs)

Insomnia

Motion sickness

Vertigo

SIDE EFFECTS
SEE ANTIHISTAMINES.

DONG QUAI

LATIN NAME
Angelica sinensis

VITAL STATISTICS

GENERAL DESCRIPTION

Also known as Chinese angelica root, dong quai is used by Chinese herbalists as a treatment for several gynecological complaints. Modern acupuncturists sometimes also inject the herb into acupuncture points to treat pain, especially that from neuralgia and arthritis. Look for a long, moist, oily plant as the source of the root, which has brown bark and a white cross section. This fragrant herb is characterized as sweet, acrid, bitter, and warm, according to traditional Chinese medicine.

Chinese medicine takes a holistic approach to healthcare, fashioning remedies to treat the entire being as well as the specific parts or areas. Single herbs may be used alone or in combination with other herbs to prevent and combat disease, which is thought to arise from disturbances in the flow of a bodily energy called chi (pronounced "chee") and blood, or from a lack of balance in the complementary states of yin and yang.

PREPARATIONS

This root is widely available in bulk and in tablet form at Chinese pharmacies, Asian markets, and Western health food stores. You should avoid the herb if it is dry or has a greenish brown cross section. Frying the herb in vinegar or wine improves its tonic effect on blood circulation. Toasting it to ash increases its ability to stop bleeding.

COMBINATIONS: Mixed with astragalus, dong quai provides a tonic for treating fatigue and other symptoms associated with loss of blood. A blend of dong quai, white peony root, Chinese foxglove root cooked in wine, and cnidium root (Ligusticum chuanxiong) is prescribed for menstrual irregularity and similar conditions. Dong quai is also combined with honeysuckle flowers and red peony root to form a preparation that reduces the swelling and alleviates the pain of abscesses and sores.

Consult a Chinese medicine practitioner for further information on mixtures and doses.

PRECAUTIONS

SPECIAL INFORMATION

- You should not take dong quai during the early stages of pregnancy.
- Check on the use of this herb with your Chinese medicine practitioner if you have diarrhea or abdominal bloating; it is not recommended in some cases.

TARGET AILMENTS

Take internally for:

Menstrual irregularity; lack of menstruation; painful or insubstantial menstruation; stabbing pain; pain caused by traumatic injury; poor blood circulation; pale complexion; possible anemia; carbuncles that, according to traditional Chinese medicine, arise from stagnant blood; abscesses; sores; lightheadedness; blurred vision; heart palpitations

SIDE EFFECTS

NONE EXPECTED IF USED AS DIRECTED.

ECHINACEA

LATIN NAME
Echinacea spp.

VITAL STATISTICS

GENERAL DESCRIPTION

Herbalists value the dried root of echinacea for its broad-based action against many types of viral and bacterial illnesses such as colds, bronchitis, ear infections, influenza, and cystitis. Laboratory testing shows that it contains echinacoside, an ingredient that may have antibiotic effects. Another ingredient, echinacein, is believed to block some mechanisms that enable infectious viruses or bacteria to invade body tissue.

In the laboratory, echinacea seems to bolster white blood cells in their battle against foreign microorganisms; it may increase the production of T cells, which join other white blood cells in the fight against infectious agents. Echinacea can also be effective topically for eczema and other skin problems.

PREPARATIONS
Over the counter:
Available in dried form in bulk, and in teas, capsules, and tinctures.

At home:
TEA: Boil 2 tsp dried root in 1 cup water and simmer covered for 15 minutes. Drink three times a day.
COMBINATIONS: Use echinacea with yarrow or uva ursi to treat cystitis.
Consult a practitioner for the dosage appropriate for you and the specific ailment.

PRECAUTIONS

SPECIAL INFORMATION
- Do not use for more than a few weeks.
- Do not give to children younger than two at all or to older ones for more than seven to 10 days except in conjunction with a healthcare practitioner; start with minimal doses for older children and older adults.
- Check with your doctor before using echinacea if you are pregnant or nursing.

POSSIBLE INTERACTIONS
Combining echinacea with other herbs may necessitate a lower dosage.

TARGET AILMENTS

Take internally for:

Colds, the flu, and other respiratory illnesses; mononucleosis

Ear infections

Septicemia (blood poisoning)

Bladder infections

Apply externally for:

Cuts; burns; wounds

Abscesses; boils

Insect bites and stings

Hives; eczema

Herpes

SIDE EFFECTS
NONE EXPECTED

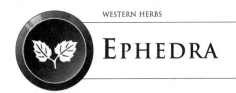

EPHEDRA

LATIN NAME
Ephedra sinica

VITAL STATISTICS

GENERAL DESCRIPTION
The roots and aboveground parts of this herb are used by Western practitioners as a bronchial decongestant and as a remedy for asthma, hay fever, and the common cold. One of its three active ingredients, ephedrine, opens the bronchial passages; this activates the heart, increasing blood pressure and speeding up metabolism. For this reason, herbalists warn that excessive use of ephedra can lead to nervousness, insomnia, and high blood pressure. In the United States, several states have set restrictions on the strength of over-the-counter products containing ephedra.

PREPARATIONS
Over the counter:
Available as fluidextract, tablets, and dried bulk herb.

At home:
TEA: Simmer covered 1 to 2 tsp ephedra with 1 cup water for 10 to 15 minutes. Drink up to 2 cups a day.
Consult a qualified practitioner for the dosage appropriate for you and your specific condition.

PRECAUTIONS

☠ WARNING
Do not take ephedra if you are pregnant or have heart disease, diabetes, glaucoma, high blood pressure, anxiety, or hyperthyroidism.
Several weight-loss aids contain ephedra. Its effectiveness derives from its accelerating effect on the metabolism, considered an unwanted side effect; thus, many healthcare professionals warn against using it to lose weight.

If you are taking any medication, consult your physician before using this herb.
This herb should not be used with children unless it is specifically prescribed by a healthcare practitioner who is knowledgeable about herbs. In any case, do not administer to children under age two. Use low-strength prescriptions for adults over 65.
Because ephedra can cause a number of side effects—and in rare cases, death—consult a practitioner before using it.

POSSIBLE INTERACTIONS
Combining ephedra with other herbs may necessitate a lower dosage.

TARGET AILMENTS
Colds; influenza; nasal and chest congestion

Asthma; hay fever

SIDE EFFECTS

NOT SERIOUS
- Insomnia
- Dry mouth
- Nervousness; irritability
- Headache; dizziness

DECREASE DOSE. CALL YOUR DOCTOR IF THESE EFFECTS PERSIST.

SERIOUS
- Increased blood pressure
- Increased heart rate
- Heart palpitations

STOP USING EPHEDRA IMMEDIATELY AND CONSULT YOUR DOCTOR.

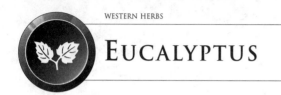

EUCALYPTUS

LATIN NAME
Eucalyptus globulus

VITAL STATISTICS

GENERAL DESCRIPTION
Native to Australia and a favorite meal for koalas, the eucalyptus tree is sometimes called the Australian fever tree or gum tree. The oil extracted from eucalyptus leaves is an important ingredient in over-the-counter mouthwashes and decongestants. Herbalists include small amounts of the oil in several preparations, including gargles for sore throat, topical antiseptics for skin injuries, rubs for arthritis, and inhalants for asthma, bronchitis, and other respiratory conditions.

PREPARATIONS
Over the counter:
Available in dry bulk, tinctures, and oils.

At home:
INHALANT: Put 1 to 3 drops of the oil in a bowl and add 1 pt boiling water; inhale steam until the vapors disappear.
ANTISEPTIC: Dilute the oil with an equal amount of an alcohol-based topical antiseptic and apply to cuts and other open wounds after you have washed them with soap.
RUB: Mix 1 to 5 drops eucalyptus oil with 1 cup olive oil.
Consult a qualified practitioner for the dosage appropriate for your specific condition.

SIDE EFFECTS

NOT SERIOUS
• Skin rash

THIS SYMPTOM MAY OCCUR WITH
EXTERNAL USE. IF IT DOES,
DISCONTINUE USE.

PRECAUTIONS

☠ WARNING
The oil of eucalyptus in concentrated form is poisonous if you ingest it. A teaspoonful can be fatal. Call your doctor immediately if you experience stomach upset or diarrhea with any dosage.

Do not administer internally to children under two years of age. For older children and older adults, start with minimal doses.

If you apply the oil to broken, irritated skin, use small amounts.

Close your eyes when inhaling eucalyptus in any form because the fumes are very powerful, and be especially careful to protect your eyes from any contact with the oils.

POSSIBLE INTERACTIONS
Combining eucalyptus with other herbs may necessitate a lower dosage.

TARGET AILMENTS
Apply externally for:
Arthritis; rheumatism
Minor cuts and scrapes
Use as an inhalant in an extremely dilute form for:
Asthma
Colds, flu, and other respiratory illnesses
Bronchitis
Whooping cough

EVENING PRIMROSE OIL

LATIN NAME
Oenothera biennis

VITAL STATISTICS

GENERAL INFORMATION

Herbalists recommend the oil from the seeds of the plant known as evening primrose for a wide range of ailments that includes arthritis and premenstrual syndrome. Evening primrose supplements may also benefit brittle hair and fingernails, and may help to keep dry eyes lubricated. Native Americans and early settlers in North America used the oil to treat asthma, gastrointestinal ills, and bruises.

The therapeutic component of evening primrose oil, known as gamma-linolenic acid (GLA), is an essential fatty acid that the Western diet often lacks. GLA supports the body's production of hormones known as prostaglandins, which affect the body's hormone balance. When the body's supply of essential fatty acids such as GLA is deficient, the effects of premenstrual syndrome, diabetes, and other disorders may become more pronounced.

Evening primrose oil may also, through its anti-inflammatory action, be useful in treating sore breasts in nursing mothers. In addition, recent studies suggest that evening primrose oil may have an anticlotting action. Some herbalists believe that this property may make the oil helpful in the treatment of coronary artery disease.

PREPARATIONS

Available in capsules and in liquid form. Consult a qualified practitioner for the dosage appropriate for you and the specific condition being treated.

PRECAUTIONS

SPECIAL INFORMATION

- Evening primrose supplements must be taken regularly for at least a month before their beneficial effects can be noticed.
- Consult a practitioner before using evening primrose oil medicinally for children.

TARGET AILMENTS

Premenstrual syndrome

Arthritis

Dry eyes

Multiple sclerosis

High blood pressure

Eczema

Brittle hair and fingernails

SIDE EFFECTS

NOT SERIOUS

- Headache
- Skin rash
- Nausea

LOWER YOUR DOSAGE OR DISCONTINUE USE ALTOGETHER.

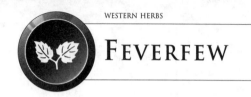

FEVERFEW

LATIN NAME
Tanacetum parthenium
(or Chrysanthemum
parthenium)

VITAL STATISTICS

GENERAL DESCRIPTION
Feverfew is a perennial with small, daisylike blossoms and leaves that are medicinal. In the late 1970s, British researchers found feverfew leaves helpful in treating migraine headaches where other treatments had failed. They believe this relief is due to the chemical parthenolide, which blocks the release of inflammatory substances from the blood. The researchers consider these inflammatory elements, which affect the walls of the brain's blood vessels, to be key components in the onset of a migraine.

You may need to take feverfew daily for two to three months before it has any effect.

PREPARATIONS
Over the counter:
Available in dry bulk, pills, capsules, and tinctures.

At home:
Chew two fresh or frozen leaves a day for migraines. If you find the leaves too bitter, substitute capsules or pills containing 85 mg of the leaf material, but fresh leaves are best for immediate results.

TEA: Steep covered 2 tsp dried herb in 1 cup boiling water for 5 to 10 minutes; drink 2 to 3 cups per day.
Consult a qualified practitioner for the dosage appropriate for you and the specific condition being treated.

PRECAUTIONS

SPECIAL INFORMATION
- Do not use feverfew if you are pregnant; it may stimulate uterine contractions.
- Feverfew may interfere with the blood's clotting ability; talk to your doctor before using if you have a clotting disorder or take anticoagulant medicine.
- Use of this herb by children for more than seven to 10 days should be done in conjunction with a healthcare practitioner.

POSSIBLE INTERACTIONS
Combining feverfew with other herbs may necessitate a lower dosage.

TARGET AILMENTS
Migraine headaches

SIDE EFFECTS

SERIOUS
- Internal mouth sores
- Abdominal pain

CHEWING FRESH OR DRIED FEVERFEW MAY CAUSE THESE SYMPTOMS. IF THEY DEVELOP, DISCONTINUE USE AND NOTIFY YOUR DOCTOR IMMEDIATELY.

FIBER, DIETARY

VITAL STATISTICS

DAILY DOSAGE
30 grams

GENERAL DESCRIPTION
Dietary fiber is the part of whole grains, fruits, and vegetables that remains undigested as it travels through the alimentary canal. Soluble fiber, such as that found in oat bran, beans, apples, and carrots, helps lower blood cholesterol. Insoluble fiber, such as that found in wheat bran, rice bran, and lentils, is especially helpful for adding bulk to improve digestion and prevent constipation. Most nutritionists favor food sources, but several over-the-counter supplements are available, such as psyllium seed for constipation.

NATURAL SOURCES
Good sources are fresh fruits and vegetables, nuts and seeds, and whole-grain foods.

PREPARATIONS
Available as psyllium seed, oat bran and rice bran, glucomannan, guar gum, or fennel seed.

Supplements are available as capsules, tablets, oral suspension, flakes, or wafers.

To help relieve constipation, mix bran with fruit juice or cereal. Start with 1 tbsp a day and gradually increase to 3 to 4 tbsp.

PRECAUTIONS

☠ WARNING
Consult your doctor before taking fiber supplements if you have Crohn's disease.

SPECIAL INFORMATION
- Fiber intake should be increased gradually. Supplements may cause intestinal gas, but this effect will subside as the body adjusts.
- Increase water intake when increasing dietary fiber, because fiber absorbs water.

POSSIBLE INTERACTIONS
Digoxin: decreased effectiveness.
Minerals (calcium, iron, zinc, and copper): decreased absorption of these minerals.

TARGET AILMENTS

High cholesterol

Constipation; hemorrhoids

Diverticulitis

Obesity

Heart disease

Non-insulin-dependent diabetes

Cancers of the colon and breast

SIDE EFFECTS

NOT SERIOUS
- Flatulence or bloating

SERIOUS
- Blocked colon, indicated by pain, fever, lack of bowel movements, and distended abdomen

CALL YOUR DOCTOR IMMEDIATELY.

FOLIC ACID (VITAMIN B9)

VITAL STATISTICS

OTHER NAMES
vitamin B9, folacin, folate

GENERAL DESCRIPTION
Healthy hair, skin, nails, nerves, mucous membranes, and blood all depend on folic acid—sometimes called vitamin B9, folacin, or folate. A critical component of RNA and DNA—the genetic material that controls the growth and repair of all cells—folic acid supports immune function and may help deter atherosclerosis as well as some cancers of the mucous membranes.

Extreme vitamin B9 deficiency may cause megaloblastic anemia, a disease characterized by red blood cells that are too few in number and malformed. Symptoms include headache; pallor; fatigue; loss of appetite; insomnia; diarrhea; and a red, inflamed tongue. Those who are most susceptible to folic acid deficiency include alcoholics, people with gastrointestinal diseases, adolescents who subsist mainly on junk food, women taking oral contraceptives, and pregnant women who are not taking supplements.

RDA
Men: 200 mcg
Women: 180 mcg
Women of childbearing age: 400 mcg

NATURAL SOURCES
Sources of folic acid include liver, kidneys, avocados, beans, beets, celery, eggs, fish, green leafy vegetables, nuts, seeds, peas, orange juice, and fortified breakfast cereals.

PRECAUTIONS

☠ WARNING
High doses of folic acid are not toxic but may mask the symptoms of vitamin B12 deficiency. Therefore, it's best to increase folic acid intake through diet or a multivitamin that contains low-dose folic acid, rather than through individual supplements, which have to be prescribed by a doctor.

SPECIAL INFORMATION
A healthy diet should provide adequate folic acid, but the need increases during pregnancy, with injury, with some diseases—especially cancer—and with long-term use of drugs such as aspirin and oral contraceptives. Supplements taken during pregnancy may help deter the birth defects spina bifida and cleft palate. For this reason, experts now recommend that all women of childbearing age consume 400 mcg daily.

TARGET AILMENTS
Cancer
Heart disease
Immune problems
Skin problems

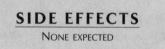

SIDE EFFECTS
NONE EXPECTED

GARLIC

LATIN NAME
Allium sativum

VITAL STATISTICS

GENERAL DESCRIPTION

Worn or carried as a protective talisman throughout the ages and valued as a pungent culinary spice, the garlic bulb has gained recognition as a medicinal remedy in Chinese and Western cultures. To release its therapeutic effects, it can be eaten either raw or cooked, Garlic's active ingredient is allicin, an amino acid derivative that is also responsible for the herb's pungent smell.

Western herbalists prescribe garlic for many of the same ailments as do their Chinese counterparts. It is also thought to strengthen the cardiovascular system by reducing cholesterol and lowering blood pressure. Although no conclusive evidence has been found, a string of Western studies suggest that incorporating garlic into the daily diet may lower the risk of heart disease.

PREPARATIONS

Over the counter:
Available as cloves and in tablet form.

At home:
TINCTURE: Combine 1 cup crushed cloves with 1 qt brandy. Shake daily for two weeks. Take up to 3 tbsp a day.
Consult a qualified practitioner for the dosage appropriate for you and the specific condition being treated.

PRECAUTIONS

SPECIAL INFORMATION
- Consult your practitioner before using garlic if you are pregnant.
- Garlic contains a blood-clot-preventing agent. If you have a blood-clotting disorder, consult an herbalist or a licensed healthcare professional.
- Garlic is thought to function as an adjunct treatment for cardiovascular disease. Consult your practitioner before using it in this capacity.

TARGET AILMENTS

Take internally for:

Colds; coughs; flu

High cholesterol

High blood pressure

Atherosclerosis

Digestive disorders

Bladder infection

Liver and gallbladder problems

Apply externally for:

Athlete's foot; ringworm

Minor skin infections

SIDE EFFECTS

NOT SERIOUS

PEOPLE ALLERGIC TO GARLIC MAY DEVELOP A RASH FROM TOUCHING OR EATING THE HERB.

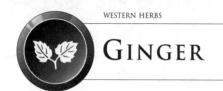

GINGER

LATIN NAME
Zingiber officinale

VITAL STATISTICS

GENERAL DESCRIPTION

Characterized by delicate yellow blooms rimmed with purple, ginger not only is a valued culinary seasoning but also is considered in many cultures to be a remedy for a range of ailments. Discovered by practitioners of traditional Ayurvedic (Hindu) medicine, gingerroot was originally thought of as a digestive aid. Today both Chinese and Western herbalists believe it relieves motion sickness and dizziness and improves digestion. Ginger is also believed to alleviate menstrual cramps. Its active constituents are gingerols, which soothe the abdomen and relieve excess gas. Some studies show that ginger may help prevent heart disease and strokes by reducing internal blood clotting and blood pressure.

PREPARATIONS

Over the counter:

Ginger is available as fresh or dried root, liquid extract, tablets, capsules, or prepared tea.

At home:

COMBINATIONS: For vomiting, ginger is mixed with pinellia root; when there is also severe abdominal pain, the herb is combined with licorice or galanga. A preparation of ginger and chamomile is used to treat menstrual irregularity. For coughing and headaches, ginger is mixed with dried bamboo.

TEA: Simmer 1 to 2 tsp dried gingerroot in 1 cup water for 5 to 10 minutes.

Consult a qualified practitioner for the dosage appropriate for you and the specific condition being treated.

PRECAUTIONS

☠ WARNING

If you are pregnant, consult a herbalist or a licensed healthcare professional before using.

POSSIBLE INTERACTIONS

Combining ginger with other herbs may necessitate a lower dosage.

TARGET AILMENTS
Motion sickness
Morning sickness
Digestive disorders
Menstrual cramps
Colds; flu
Arthritis
Elevated cholesterol level
High blood pressure

SIDE EFFECTS

NOT SERIOUS

- Heartburn

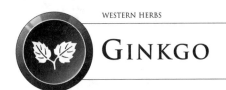

GINKGO

LATIN NAME
Ginkgo biloba

VITAL STATISTICS

GENERAL INFORMATION

Chinese herbalists have used the leaves of the ginkgo tree for thousands of years to treat asthma, chilblains, and swellings. Today, Western herbalists value ginkgo leaves for their action against vascular diseases that typically affect the elderly. One of ginkgo's most important benefits is its ability to increase vasodilation (expansion of blood vessels) and thereby improve blood flow in capillaries and arteries, especially in peripheral areas such as the lower legs and feet. It also appears to improve blood flow to the brain, decreasing symptoms such as dizziness and memory loss.

Ginkgo may also help reduce retinal damage from macular degeneration, a cause of blindness particularly threatening for diabetics. And it may help reverse deafness caused by reduced blood flow to the auditory nerves.

PREPARATIONS

Ginkgo leaves are available in dry bulk, capsules, or tincture. You can find a standardized product known as ginkgo biloba extract (GBE) in health food stores. Most herbalists recommend using only OTC ginkgo products.

PRECAUTIONS

SPECIAL INFORMATION

- Some people are unable to tolerate ginkgo, even in small doses.
- Do not use if you have a clotting disorder, or if you are pregnant or nursing.
- This herb should not be used with children unless specifically prescribed by a healthcare practitioner knowledgeable about herbs.
- Use in medicinal amounts only in consultation with a healthcare professional.

POSSIBLE INTERACTIONS

Combining ginkgo with other herbs may necessitate a lower dosage.

TARGET AILMENTS

Vertigo; tinnitus

Alzheimer's disease

Phlebitis; leg ulcers

Cerebral atherosclerosis

Diabetic vascular disease

Raynaud's syndrome

Headache; depression

In the elderly, lack of concentration or mental and emotional fatigue

Clotting disorders, including strokes and heart attacks

SIDE EFFECTS

SERIOUS

- Irritability; restlessness
- Diarrhea; nausea; vomiting

IF THESE SYMPTOMS DEVELOP, CHECK WITH YOUR PRACTITIONER TO SEE IF YOU SHOULD LOWER YOUR DOSAGE OR STOP TAKING GINKGO COMPLETELY.

GINSENG, ASIAN

LATIN NAME
Panax ginseng

VITAL STATISTICS

GENERAL DESCRIPTION

Asian ginseng, considered the most potent form of ginseng, strengthens the immune system and increases the body's ability to deal with fatigue and stress. Today herbalists prescribe Asian ginseng root for minor ailments such as fever, colds, coughs, and menstrual irregularities.

PRECAUTIONS

☠ WARNING

If you have any of the following conditions, use ginseng only under the direction of a herbalist or a licensed healthcare professional: pregnancy, insomnia, hay fever, fibrocystic breasts, asthma, emphysema, high blood pressure, blood-clotting problems, heart disorders, diabetes. This herb should not be used with children unless specifically prescribed by a healthcare practitioner knowledgeable about herbs.

PREPARATIONS

Over the counter:
Ginseng is available as fresh or dried root, root powder, capsules, tablets, prepared tea, freeze-dried root, and cured rock candy.

At home:
CHINESE: Boil fresh roots, covered, in water for 3 to 7 minutes. Prick roots with needles. Dry roots in the sun and then soak in thick sugar 10 to 12 hours.
WESTERN: TEA: Boil covered 1 tbsp fresh root with 1 cup water for 15 to 20 minutes. Drink up to 2 cups a day.
Consult a qualified practitioner for the dosage appropriate for your specific condition.

TARGET AILMENTS

Take internally (Chinese) for:

Symptoms of shock
Profuse sweating
Ice-cold extremities
Shortness of breath
Fever; thirst
Irritability
Diarrhea, vomiting
Distention of the abdomen

Take internally (Western) for:

Depression
Fatigue; stress
Colds; influenza
Respiratory problems
Inflammation
Damaged immune system

SIDE EFFECTS

NOT SERIOUS

- Headache
- Insomnia or anxiety
- Breast soreness
- Skin rashes

CALL YOUR DOCTOR IF THESE EFFECTS PERSIST.

SERIOUS

- Asthma attacks
- Increased blood pressure
- Heart palpitations
- Postmenopausal bleeding

STOP USING GINSENG AND CONSULT YOUR DOCTOR.

GLUCOSAMINE SULFATE

VITAL STATISTICS

GENERAL DESCRIPTION

Glucosamine is a natural compound that plays a role in forming bones, nails, tendons, skin, and ligaments. It also acts to maintain and repair the cartilage surrounding bone joints. It's considered the building block of this cartilage. Glucosamine sulfate is an artificially synthesized substance made up of glucose, nitrogen, hydrogen, and sulfur.

Studies in Europe and in Japan suggest that glucosamine sulfate can be effective in treating at least one type of arthritis, osteoarthritis. Osteoarthritis develops when the cartilage around the joints breaks down. The joints gradually deteriorate and become painful and stiff. In one study in Italy, osteoarthritis patients treated with injectable glucosamine sulfate, followed by an oral form of the supplement, reported relief from pain at rest and pain during movement. Another study showed that osteoarthritis patients' pain, joint tenderness, and swelling were relieved after six to eight weeks of treatment with glucosamine sulfate.

The supplement is believed to work by stimulating cells to synthesize proteoglycans and glycosaminoglycans, two substances that play a role in building cartilage. Proponents of glucosamine sulfate say the supplement also has anti-inflammatory qualities, but without the potentially dangerous side effects associated with aspirin and nonsteroidal anti-inflammatory drugs (NSAIDs).

Critics say none of the studies to date have shown any long-term benefits of glucosamine sulfate, either for relieving symptoms or for preventing further deterioration of the cartilage and the joints. They also argue there is little known about any potential long-term side effects.

PREPARATIONS

Glucosamine sulfate is sold in the United States in capsule form as a dietary supplement.

PRECAUTIONS

SPECIAL INFORMATION

Some books and media reports have touted glucosamine sulfate as a cure for osteoarthritis, but experts warn consumers not to rely on the supplement as a treatment for the disease. They advise checking with a physician for advice on effective lifestyle changes and proven treatments.

TARGET AILMENTS
Joint pain
Joint stiffness
Osteoarthritis

SIDE EFFECTS

NOT SERIOUS
- Stomach upset; heartburn; diarrhea; nausea; indigestion

CALL YOUR DOCTOR IF THESE SYMPTOMS PERSIST.

GOLDENSEAL

LATIN NAME
Hydrastis canadensis

VITAL STATISTICS

GENERAL INFORMATION

Herbalists use goldenseal to treat several respiratory and skin infections. The herb acts as a stimulant and seems to affect the body's mucous membranes by drying up secretions, reducing inflammation, and fighting infection through the mild antimicrobial action of its active ingredient, berberine. Goldenseal also aids digestion by promoting the production of digestive enzymes. In addition it may control postpartum bleeding by its astringent action.

PREPARATIONS

Over the counter:
Available in dry bulk, capsules, and tincture.

At home:
TEA: Pour 1 cup boiling water onto 2 tsp goldenseal; steep covered for 10 to 15 minutes. Drink three times daily.
DOUCHE: Simmer covered 1 tbsp powdered herb in 1 pt water for 10 minutes. The liquid should be as warm as is tolerable. Douche daily, up to two weeks.
Consult a practitioner for the dosage appropriate for you and your specific condition.

SIDE EFFECTS

NOT SERIOUS

IN HIGH DOSES, GOLDENSEAL CAN IRRITATE THE SKIN, MOUTH, THROAT, AND VAGINA. IT MAY ALSO CAUSE NAUSEA AND DIARRHEA. IF ANY OF THESE DEVELOP, STOP TAKING IMMEDIATELY.

PRECAUTIONS

SPECIAL INFORMATION

- Do not use goldenseal if you are pregnant.
- Do not use without consulting a physician if you have had heart disease, diabetes, glaucoma, a stroke, or high blood pressure.
- Do not give to children under two; give small doses to older ones and adults over 65. Use by children for more than seven days should be monitored by a healthcare practitioner.

POSSIBLE INTERACTIONS

Combining goldenseal with other herbs may necessitate a lower dosage.

TARGET AILMENTS

Take internally for:

Infectious diarrhea; gastritis

Ulcers; gallstones; jaundice

Sinusitis; ear infections

Laryngitis; sore throat

Infected gums

Postpartum uterine bleeding

Vaginal yeast infections

Apply externally for:

Eczema; impetigo

Ringworm; athlete's foot

Contact dermatitis

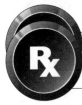

GUAIFENESIN

VITAL STATISTICS

DRUG CLASS
Expectorants

BRAND NAMES
Rx: Entex LA
OTC: Primatene Dual Action Formula, Robitussin-CF, Robitussin-DM, Triaminic Expectorant, Vicks DayQuil LiquiCaps, Vicks DayQuil Liquid

GENERAL DESCRIPTION
Guaifenesin is an expectorant drug, used to provide symptomatic relief from coughs, particularly those associated with the common cold or flu. The medication works by thinning and loosening mucus or phlegm from the upper respiratory tract, making it easier to cough up and expel the secretions.

This drug is used in many over-the-counter and prescription cough preparations, often in combination with a decongestant, an antihistamine, or some other medication. Guaifenesin is available in tablet, capsule, or liquid form.

PRECAUTIONS

SPECIAL INFORMATION
- If you are using the extended-release tablet form of this medication, swallow it whole; do not crush or chew the tablet before swallowing it.
- This medication is most effective when taken on an empty stomach.
- To help guaifenesin loosen mucus from the lungs, drink eight to 10 glasses of fluid each day, including a glass of water after each dose.

- If you are pregnant or nursing, check with your doctor before using this medication.
- Do not give this medication to a child under the age of two without first consulting the child's pediatrician.
- Do not take this drug for persistent cough due to smoking, asthma, bronchitis, or emphysema.
- If your cough does not improve within seven days, see your doctor.

POSSIBLE INTERACTIONS
None expected.

TARGET AILMENTS

Coughs due to the common cold, flu, and other minor upper respiratory conditions

SIDE EFFECTS

NOT SERIOUS
- Stomach pain
- Diarrhea
- Nausea
- Drowsiness
- Mild weakness

CONTACT YOUR DOCTOR IF THESE SYMPTOMS PERSIST OR BECOME BOTHERSOME.

SERIOUS
- Skin rash
- Persistent headache
- Vomiting
- High fever

CONTACT YOUR DOCTOR AT ONCE.

HIBISCUS

LATIN NAME
Hibiscus sabdariffa

VITAL STATISTICS

GENERAL INFORMATION

Hibiscus, a widespread category of annuals whose lush, showy flowers are nearly synonymous with tropical beauty, includes more than 200 species of plants. Most of them are believed to have some medicinal properties; different species are used in Ayurvedic (Hindu), Chinese, and Western herbal medicines. *Hibiscus sabdariffa,* also known as roselle or Jamaica sorrel, is valued for its mild laxative effect and for its ability to increase urination, attributed to two diuretic ingredients, ascorbic acid and glycolic acid. Because it contains citric acid, a refrigerant, it is used as a cooling herb, providing relief during hot weather by increasing the flow of blood to the skin's surface and dilating the pores to cool the skin.

Hibiscus seeds, leaves, fruits, and roots are used in various folk remedies, and tea is made from the flowers, in particular the calyx, the leaflike segment that makes up the outermost part of the flower. Its flowers are also used in jams and jellies to impart a tart, refreshing taste. The tart flavor of hibiscus tea may clash with that of other strong-tasting herbs, such as chamomile or dandelion; mix with mint or rose hip tea instead.

PREPARATIONS
Over the counter:
Fresh or dried hibiscus flowers and teas are available in health food stores.

At home:
TEA: Use 2 tsp crumbled dried blossom or 1 tbsp fresh chopped blossom per cup of boiling water; steep covered 10 minutes. Drink up to 3 cups per day. Iced hibiscus tea is also refreshing.

Consult a qualified practitioner for the dosage appropriate for you and the specific condition being treated.

PRECAUTIONS

SPECIAL INFORMATION

Because many types of hibiscus are sold, check with an herbal practitioner to determine if the species you are using is an appropriate treatment. Some species may not be recommended for pregnant women.

POSSIBLE INTERACTIONS

Combining hibiscus with other herbs may necessitate a lower dosage.

TARGET AILMENTS

Take internally for:

Constipation

Mild bladder infections

Mild nausea

Apply the herb or extract externally for:

Sunburn

SIDE EFFECTS

NOT SERIOUS

YOU MIGHT NOTICE A SLIGHTLY DRY SENSATION IN THE MOUTH, WHICH IS CAUSED BY THE HERB'S ASTRINGENT PROPERTY.

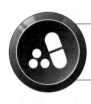

HYDROCORTISONE

VITAL STATISTICS

DRUG CLASS
Corticosteroids

BRAND NAMES
Cortaid, Cortizone

OTHER DRUGS IN THIS CLASS
Rx: beclomethasone, betamethasone, fluticasone, methylprednisolone, mometasone furoate, prednisone, triamcinolone

GENERAL DESCRIPTION
Hydrocortisone cream is used for temporary relief of minor skin problems, including inflammation and rashes caused by eczema, poison ivy, poison oak, poison sumac, insect bites, psoriasis, soaps, detergents, cosmetics, and jewelry. The drug treats only the symptoms, not the underlying causes.

Like other corticosteroids, hydrocortisone is a powerful drug. It can affect almost all parts of the body, so it should be used with caution. For more information, see Corticosteroids.

TARGET AILMENTS

Rash

Inflammation

Itching

Psoriasis

Eczema

Sunburn

PRECAUTIONS

SPECIAL INFORMATION
- Hydrocortisone should not be used for rosacea, acne, viral skin infections such as herpes, or fungal infections such as athlete's foot.
- Do not use this medication near your eyes; with prolonged use, doing so can cause a number of problems, including glaucoma or cataracts.
- If you have diabetes, check with your doctor before using hydrocortisone.
- These creams may sting slightly when they are first applied.
- Do not use excessive quantities of this medication or bind dressings tightly over the treated area.
- Corticosteroid topical creams may be absorbed into your system after prolonged use. Tell your doctor if you are taking any other medication and watch for any significant side effects or possible drug interactions.
- Hydrocortisone should be used with caution if you are allergic to other corticosteroids; if you have an infection or thin skin at the treatment site; or if you have or have had cataracts, glaucoma, diabetes, or tuberculosis.
- Ask your doctor about the risks and benefits of corticosteroid treatment if you have or have had any of the following conditions: HIV infection or AIDS, heart disease, hypertension, ulcerative colitis, diabetes, diverticulitis, gastritis or peptic ulcers, recent chickenpox or measles, candidiasis or other fungal infections, glaucoma, herpes simplex, liver or kidney disease, myasthenia gravis, osteoporosis, anastomoses, lupus, tuberculosis, recent intestinal problems, or any infection, such as a cold or flu.
- One of the actions of corticosteroids is to

CONTINUED

HYDROCORTISONE

suppress your immune system, thereby making you more susceptible to opportunistic infections. Corticosteroids can also mask symptoms of infection that occur while you are taking the drugs; because the symptoms will not appear, an infection may worsen without your being aware of it.

- Prolonged use of corticosteroids can cause birth defects. Pregnant and nursing women should avoid these drugs.
- Prolonged use of corticosteroids increases the risk of osteoporosis, cataracts, glaucoma, Cushing's syndrome (moon face), and diabetes. It can also reactivate tuberculosis.
- Check with your doctor before you stop using corticosteroids. It may be necessary to reduce the dosage gradually to avoid serious consequences.

SIDE EFFECTS

NOT SERIOUS

- Mild and transient skin rash
- Burning
- Irritation
- Dryness
- Redness
- Itchiness
- Scaling

CALL YOUR DOCTOR IF THESE SYMPTOMS PERSIST OR BECOME BOTHERSOME.

SERIOUS

- Eye pain
- Loss of or blurred vision
- Stomach pain or burning
- Black, tarry stools
- Severe and lasting skin rash, hives, or burning, itching, or painful skin
- Blisters, acne, or other skin problems
- Nausea or vomiting
- High blood pressure
- Foot or leg swelling
- Rapid weight gain
- Fluid retention (edema)
- Prolonged sore throat, fever, cold, or other signs of infection

CONTACT YOUR DOCTOR IMMEDIATELY.

IBUPROFEN

VITAL STATISTICS

DRUG CLASS
Analgesics [Nonsteroidal Anti-Inflammatory Drugs (NSAIDs)]

BRAND NAMES
Rx: Children's Motrin Ibuprofen Suspension, various forms of Motrin for adults
OTC: Advil, Advil Cold and Sinus, Children's Motrin Ibuprofen Suspension, Midol-200, Motrin IB, Nuprin, Pamprin

GENERAL DESCRIPTION
Introduced in 1969, ibuprofen became available for the over-the-counter (OTC) market in 1984. The drug is used to relieve headaches, menstrual cramps, muscle aches, rheumatoid arthritis, osteoarthritis, and minor aches and pains of the common cold. It also reduces inflammation and fever. This drug is used by people who cannot take aspirin, or when acetaminophen or aspirin is not effective. For further information, see Nonsteroidal Anti-Inflammatory Drugs (NSAIDs).

TARGET AILMENTS

Inflammation, especially related to arthritis

Pain, especially from inflammation, dental and other surgeries, menstruation, and migraines

Fever

PRECAUTIONS

☠ WARNING
Do not take ibuprofen during the last three months of pregnancy.

SPECIAL INFORMATION
- Do not use ibuprofen if allergic to NSAIDs or to aspirin. It may cause bronchoconstriction or anaphylaxis in aspirin-sensitive asthmatics.
- Avoid this drug or consult your doctor before using it if you have asthma, peptic ulcer, enteritis, heart disease, high blood pressure, bleeding problems, or liver or kidney impairment.

SIDE EFFECTS

- Dizziness, drowsiness, or headache
- Mild abdominal pain; constipation or diarrhea; heartburn or nausea

CONSULT YOUR DOCTOR IF THESE SYMPTOMS PERSIST.

SERIOUS
- Anaphylactic reaction (hives, rash, intense itching, and trouble breathing)
- Gastrointestinal bleeding; ulceration; stomach perforation (black or tarry stools)
- Angina; irregular heartbeat
- Diminished hearing or ringing in the ears
- Fluid retention
- Jaundice; blood in urine

CALL YOUR DOCTOR IMMEDIATELY.

IODINE

VITAL STATISTICS

GENERAL DESCRIPTION

Iodine was one of the first minerals recognized as essential to human health. For centuries, it has been known to prevent and treat goiter—enlargement of the thyroid gland. As part of several thyroid hormones, iodine strongly influences nutrient metabolism; nerve and muscle function; skin, hair, tooth, and nail condition; and physical and mental development. Iodine may also help convert beta carotene into vitamin A, and it is an effective antiseptic and water sterilizer.

Iodine deficiency is now uncommon; besides goiter, the effects of deficiency include weight gain, hair loss, listlessness, insomnia, and some forms of mental retardation.

RDA
Adults: 150 mcg
Pregnant women: 175 mcg

NATURAL SOURCES

Kelp, seafood, and vegetables grown in iodine-rich soils are excellent sources of this mineral. More than half of all the salt consumed in the United States is iodized, supplying sufficient iodine in a regular diet.

PRECAUTIONS

SPECIAL INFORMATION

- Supplements are usually unnecessary, but pregnant women should ensure sufficient intake for themselves and their babies to prevent potential mental retardation or cretinism, a form of dwarfism in infants.
- Most excess iodine is excreted by the kidneys, but an extremely high intake may cause nervousness, hyperactivity, headache, rashes, a metallic taste in the mouth, and goiter—in this case due to hyperactivity of the thyroid gland.
- In rare cases, iodine may inhibit thyroid hormone secretion.

TARGET AILMENTS

Goiter

Skin problems

SIDE EFFECTS
NONE EXPECTED

IRON

VITAL STATISTICS

GENERAL DESCRIPTION

Iron is found in hemoglobin, the protein in red blood cells that transports oxygen from the lungs to body tissues. It is also a component of myoglobin, a protein that provides extra fuel to muscles during exertion.

Lack of iron deprives body tissues of oxygen and may cause iron deficiency anemia; warning signs include fatigue, paleness, dizziness, sensitivity to cold, listlessness, irritability, poor concentration, and heart palpitations. Because iron strengthens immune function, iron deficiency also may increase susceptibility to infection. Women need more iron before menopause than after, because menstruation causes iron loss each month.

On a doctor's recommendation, adults can augment their iron intake by means of a multinutrient supplement. Straight iron supplements should be taken only under a doctor's supervision.

RDA
Adults: 10 mg
Premenopausal women: 15 mg
Pregnant women: 30 mg

NATURAL SOURCES
Dietary iron exists in two forms: heme iron, found in red meat, chicken, seafood, and other animal products; and nonheme iron, found in dark green vegetables, whole grains, nuts, dried fruit, blackstrap molasses, and other plant foods. Many flour-based food products are fortified with iron. Heme iron is easier to absorb, but eating foods containing nonheme iron along with foods that have heme iron or vitamin C will maximize iron absorption.

PRECAUTIONS

☠ WARNING

Though uncommon, severe iron poisoning can result in coma, heart failure, and death.

Children should never be given adult iron supplements. If your pediatrician recommends an iron supplement, make sure it is a specific, child-formulated variety.

SPECIAL INFORMATION
- Coffee, tea, soy-based foods, antacids, and tetracycline inhibit iron absorption, as do excessive amounts of calcium, zinc, and manganese.
- People who have special iron-intake needs include menstruating or pregnant women, children under age two, vegetarians, and anyone with bleeding conditions such as hemorrhoids or bleeding stomach ulcers.
- Excess iron inhibits absorption of phosphorus, interferes with immune function, and may increase your risk of developing cancer, cirrhosis, or heart attack.
- Symptoms of iron toxicity include diarrhea, vomiting, headache, dizziness, fatigue, stomach cramps, and weak pulse.
- Excess iron may cause constipation.

TARGET AILMENTS

Anemia

Fatigue

SIDE EFFECTS
NONE EXPECTED

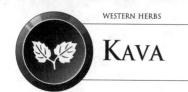

KAVA

LATIN NAME
Piper methysticum

VITAL STATISTICS

GENERAL DESCRIPTION

Drinking kava, a beverage brewed from the dried roots and rhizomes of an indigenous pepper plant, has been a feature of some South Pacific religious rituals for many centuries. Today kava is frequently prescribed, for that same euphoric effect, as an antidepressant; practitioners find it useful for treating anxiety and tension. Because of its diuretic action, it is also used to treat gout and rheumatism. In addition, kava is believed to act as an antiseptic and anti-inflammatory agent in the urinary tract, making it suitable for treating urinary tract infections such as cystitis; it is also used for prostatitis (inflammation of the prostate gland) that may arise from bacteria traveling from the urethra.

Western herbalists recommend kava for its sedative properties, which do not seem to impair mental alertness. The active ingredients, called kavalactones, act on the stem and other parts of the brain to yield kava's mild tranquilizing effect. While kava compounds do not seem to be addictive, the herb still must be used with caution.

PREPARATIONS

Available in dry bulk, capsules, and tinctures. Consult a qualified practitioner for the dosage appropriate for you and the specific condition being treated.

PRECAUTIONS

☠ WARNING

Long-term, constant use of kava in large doses has been associated with damage to the liver, skin, eyes, and even the spinal cord.

SPECIAL INFORMATION

Use of this herb by children for more than seven to 10 days should be done in conjunction with a healthcare practitioner.

POSSIBLE INTERACTIONS

Combining kava with other herbs may necessitate a lower dosage.

TARGET AILMENTS
Take internally for:
Urinary disorders
Prostate inflammations
Gout
Rheumatism
Insomnia; fatigue
Depression
Muscle spasms

SIDE EFFECTS

NOT SERIOUS

CHRONIC USE CAN CAUSE A TYPE OF DERMATITIS THAT WILL CLEAR UP WHEN YOU STOP TAKING KAVA.

SERIOUS

TOO MUCH KAVA CAN CAUSE INTOXICATION OR DROWSINESS. IF THIS HAPPENS, LOWER YOUR DOSAGE OR STOP TAKING KAVA.

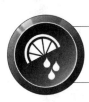

LACTOBACILLUS ACIDOPHILUS

VITAL STATISTICS

OTHER NAME
acidophilus

DAILY DOSAGE
One or two capsules twice a day before meals (or as directed)

GENERAL DESCRIPTION
Bacteria are usually something to avoid. But *Lactobacillus acidophilus* is one type of bacteria you may want to seek out. Acidophilus resembles certain bacteria that occur naturally in our bodies. These natural bacteria inhabit the colon and vagina, where they play an important role in digestion and in controlling the overgrowth of fungi and other organisms. For many people, taking antibiotics can upset this delicate balance. This is because antibiotics cannot distinguish between "good" bacteria and harmful bacteria. When populations of "helpful" bacteria diminish, the result can be intestinal problems and, for women, vaginal yeast infections. Ingesting acidophilus during and after a course of antibiotics can help restore populations of good bacteria.

Acidophilus can help in other ways as well. For example, these bacteria have been found to help reduce the incidence of yeast infections in susceptible women. By helping to break down lactose (milk sugar), acidophilus can make it easier for people who are lactose intolerant to digest milk, and it may help relieve symptoms of spastic colon.

Several studies suggest that acidophilus may one day be useful in treating or reducing the risk of colon cancer. Some proponents believe that these bacteria may also help lower cholesterol levels, boost immunity, and help in the treatment of allergies, although these benefits have not been proved.

PREPARATIONS
Acidophilus is sold in capsules, tablets, powders, and liquids. It is also added to some yogurt, kefir, and milk products. Check the label carefully to make sure acidophilus is listed as an ingredient.

PRECAUTIONS

☠ WARNING
People who have serious, medically treated intestinal problems should consult their doctor before taking acidophilus.

SPECIAL INFORMATION
High temperatures can kill acidophilus. Any products containing these bacteria should be kept in the refrigerator.

TARGET AILMENTS

Canker sores

Constipation; diarrhea; indigestion; gas

Lactose intolerance; postantibiotic therapy; spastic colon

Yeast infections; urinary tract infections

SIDE EFFECTS
NONE EXPECTED

LAVENDER

LATIN NAME
Lavandula angustifolia

VITAL STATISTICS

GENERAL DESCRIPTION

This evergreen shrub, native to the Mediterranean but now grown worldwide, is the most versatile of the aromatic oils. Lavender is valued for its calming, soothing, and balancing effects. Well known for its ability to ease skin disorders, the plant is also said to have analgesic and antiseptic properties.

The flowering tops of the lavender shrub are used to produce the essential oil, which is clear or yellow green. The oil glands are easily accessible on the outside of the leaves; to release the familiar aroma, rub a flower or leaf between your fingers.

PREPARATIONS

To treat minor burns, apply the pure oil to the affected area and cover with gauze.

To relieve a tension headache, moisten your index finger with 2 drops lavender oil and rub gently over the temples, behind the ears, and across the back of the neck. The oil can also be used on small wounds and insect bites.

For larger areas, dilute the oil by mixing 15 drops with 2 tbsp vegetable or nut oil or aloe gel. This mixture can be useful in treating a variety of ailments, including skin problems, muscle or joint pain, headache, and insomnia. Nearly all complaints, except skin problems, can be relieved by simply inhaling lavender oil. Use a room diffuser to scent the air or place drops on a tissue or pillow. For a therapeutic bath, mix 10 drops lavender oil in the bathwater.

PRECAUTIONS

SPECIAL INFORMATION

- Do not apply lavender oil near the eyes.
- Buy from a reputable source. Lavender is often adulterated with other oils.
- Other species of lavender are used to produce another type of oil that is sometimes sold as lavender. This other oil has different properties, however, and will not produce the same good results.

TARGET AILMENTS

Headache; depression; stress; insomnia

Muscular and joint pain; menstrual pain

Digestive problems and nausea; colds and flu

Athlete's foot

Cuts and wounds; burns and sunburn; insect bites

Acne; eczema; dermatitis

SIDE EFFECTS

NONE EXPECTED. LAVENDER IS NONTOXIC AND NONIRRITATING.

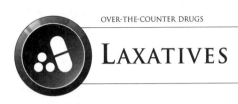

LAXATIVES

VITAL STATISTICS

GENERIC NAMES

Bulk: calcium polycarbophil, methylcellulose, psyllium hydrophilic mucilloid
Stimulant: phenolphthalein, sennosides
Stool softener: docusate

GENERAL DESCRIPTION

Laxatives are used for the temporary relief of occasional constipation and other bowel problems, and to prevent straining during bowel movements. The drugs can be taken orally in powder, liquid, granular, wafer, or pill form, or rectally as suppositories or enemas.

The bulk-forming types, considered the safest, work by absorbing water and expanding, thus increasing the moisture content of the stool to make passage easier. Increased bulk also encourages the bowels' motility. Stimulant laxatives are believed to promote evacuation by increasing peristalsis (waves of contractions) in the intestinal muscles. Stool softeners add to the bowels' liquid content, softening the stool.

PRECAUTIONS

SPECIAL INFORMATION

- If you experience a sudden change in bowel habits that lasts longer than two weeks, you should consult your doctor before using a laxative.
- If you are pregnant or nursing, consult your doctor before using any kind of laxative.
- Unless prescribed by your physician, laxatives should not be given to children under the age of six.
- Bulk-forming laxatives are best for geriatric patients with poorly functioning colons.
- Do not use laxatives if you have symptoms of appendicitis, including abdominal pain, nausea, or vomiting, or if you think you may have an intestinal obstruction.
- If you have congestive heart failure or rectal bleeding of unknown cause, do not use laxatives without your doctor's consent.
- If you are diabetic, avoid sennosides and psyllium-type laxatives that contain large amounts of sugar; instead, use sugar-free types that contain the artificial sweetener aspartame.
- If you have hypertension or are on a low-sodium diet, avoid laxatives containing sodium.
- If you have difficulty swallowing—as with dysphagia—do not take bulk-forming laxatives, which can cause an esophageal obstruction.

CONTINUED

LAXATIVES

- Chronic use of laxatives may cause excessive loss of potassium in the body.
- Laxatives can be habit forming. Use them infrequently, at the lowest effective dosage, and for no longer than one week at a time. Long-term use, particularly of stimulant laxatives, can cause physical dependence, resulting in loss of normal bowel function and chronic constipation.
- Call your doctor if the laxative fails to have the desired effect after one week of use.

POSSIBLE INTERACTIONS

Antacids, histamine H₂ blockers (cimetidine, famotidine, nizatidine, ranitidine), milk: if taken within an hour of a dosage of some types of stimulant laxatives, these medications may cause gastric upset by dissolving the outer coating of the laxative too quickly.

Laxatives that may contain danthron, mineral oil, or phenolphthalein: increased absorption of these substances, increasing the possibility of toxic effects.

Oral anticoagulants, digitalis, salicylate, tetracycline: these drugs may be less effective when taken concurrently with bulk-forming laxatives. After taking any of these medications, wait two hours before taking a laxative.

TARGET AILMENTS

Constipation

Diarrhea (bulk-forming types)

Irritable bowel syndrome, or spastic colon (bulk-forming types)

Straining during bowel movements following rectal surgery, heart attacks, childbirth, or when hemorrhoids are present

SIDE EFFECTS

NOT SERIOUS

- Harmless urine discoloration from dyes in some laxatives
- Rectal irritation (from suppositories)
- Intestinal cramping, nausea, belching, or diarrhea (from stimulant laxatives)
- Stomach cramps or throat irritation (from liquid stool softeners)

SERIOUS

- Rectal bleeding or infection (from suppositories)
- Skin rash

IF YOU DEVELOP A RASH, DISCONTINUE USE AND SEE YOUR DOCTOR.

LECITHIN

GENERAL DESCRIPTION

Lecithin is an essential natural compound found throughout the body. It's one of the main components of cell membranes, and it helps prevent these membranes from hardening. Lecithin is made up of various elements, including fatty acids, phosphorus, and choline, a B vitamin. Choline is involved in the production of the neurotransmitter acetylcholine, which is essential for the proper function of the nervous system. It is also an important component of the myelin sheaths that cover nerve fibers. Choline plays a role in processing fat and cholesterol and protects against atherosclerosis and heart disease. By emulsifying and transporting fat, choline helps to maintain the health of the liver and kidneys.

Lecithin is found in soybeans, cabbage, cauliflower, chickpeas, green beans, lentils, corn, calves' liver, and eggs. Its fat- and cholesterol-processing qualities are found only in the polyunsaturated forms of lecithin, such as those found in soybeans and vegetables. Eggs contain its saturated form. Lecithin is used as a thickener in foods such as mayonnaise, margarine, and ice cream. Most people who eat a healthy, well-balanced diet do not need to take lecithin supplements. People who take niacin or nicotinic acid for treatment of high cholesterol often are advised to take lecithin supplements because niacin can deplete the body's choline supply.

Lecithin supplements can help people with the neurological disorder tardive dyskinesia, which is characterized by involuntary, abnormal facial movements. This is a common side effect in people taking antipsychotic medications. The choline in the lecithin may help stabilize the acetylcholine neurotransmitter system in these people. Because of its role in maintaining the nervous system, lecithin supplements are being studied in combination with various drugs for treatment of Alzheimer's disease, Parkinson's disease, and Huntington's chorea, as well as Tourette's syndrome. Lecithin supplements may also be useful in preventing and treating gallstones.

PREPARATIONS

Lecithin is sold in the United States as a dietary supplement in tablet or liquid form.

TARGET AILMENTS
Dizziness; fatigue; headache
Liver disorders; high cholesterol
Bipolar depression
Insomnia
Memory loss; Alzheimer's disease

SIDE EFFECTS

SERIOUS

- Nausea; vomiting; diarrhea; bloating; abdominal pain
- Dizziness

DISCONTINUE USE AND CALL YOUR DOCTOR.

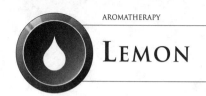

LEMON

LATIN NAME
Citrus limon

VITAL STATISTICS

GENERAL DESCRIPTION
The essential oil of lemon is pressed from the rind of the fruit. The juice is rich in vitamins A, B, and C. Lemon's healing properties make it a good all-purpose cure-all.

Probably native to Southeast Asia, the lemon tree is now cultivated worldwide. It is used extensively in the food and beverage, perfume, and pharmaceutical industries. Lemon essence is second only to orange essence in its world production and use.

PREPARATIONS
Fresh lemon oil is pale yellow, sometimes green; as it ages, it turns cloudy and brown. The oil can be applied externally and is used for a range of skin disorders and circulatory and respiratory problems.

To ease a cold or other upper respiratory discomfort, put a few drops of lemon oil on a tissue and bring the tissue to your nose to inhale. Alternatively, put a few drops on the front of the shirt the patient is wearing; this is an especially effective way to treat children's colds. Inhalation is the preparation of choice for all lemon's target ailments except skin problems.

For circulatory problems, massage the oil all over the body. Mix 6 drops lemon oil into 4 tsp almond oil to make a pleasing massage oil. For a soothing bath, add 3 to 5 drops to bathwater. Both lemon oil and lemon juice can be used internally to soothe a sore throat. The oil, however, should not be ingested. To make a gargle, add 3 drops oil to 1/2 cup warm water, or add pure lemon juice to hot water.

PRECAUTIONS

☠ WARNING
Lemon is highly phototoxic. Always dilute before using and do not apply to the skin before long periods of exposure to the sun or before entering a tanning booth.

SPECIAL INFORMATION
Lemon oil does not keep well. Check the expiration date when buying, and don't buy oil that looks cloudy.

TARGET AILMENTS
Anxiety; depression
Headache; insomnia
Throat infections, bronchitis, laryngitis, colds, and flu
High blood pressure
Varicose veins; broken capillaries
Palpitations
Dandruff; eczema; psoriasis
Premenstrual syndrome; irregular periods

SIDE EFFECTS
LEMON OIL CAN BE IRRITATING TO THE SKIN; USE IN DILUTION ONLY.

Rx LOPERAMIDE

VITAL STATISTICS

DRUG CLASS
Antidiarrheal Drugs

BRAND NAMES
Rx: Imodium
OTC: Imodium A-D

OTHER DRUGS IN THIS CLASS
attapulgite, bismuth subsalicylate

GENERAL DESCRIPTION
Introduced in 1977, loperamide is used primarily for symptomatic control of diarrhea and cramping. It is available in both over-the-counter and prescription strength. Loperamide should be taken on an empty stomach.

PRECAUTIONS

☠ WARNING
Do not use loperamide if:
- diarrhea is accompanied by high fever (101°F or higher).
- blood or mucus is present in stool.
- you have a rash or other allergic reaction to the drug.
- you are taking antibiotics or have a history of liver disease or colitis.
- you are pregnant or nursing a baby. Consult a doctor before using this drug.

POSSIBLE INTERACTIONS
Alcohol, sleeping pills, and tranquilizers: may increase depressant and sedative effects.
Antibiotics and narcotic pain medicine: may cause severe constipation if taken with antidiarrheals.

TARGET AILMENTS
Symptomatic relief of diarrhea

SIDE EFFECTS

NOT SERIOUS
- Mild constipation

CHECK WITH YOUR DOCTOR IF THE CONSTIPATION CONTINUES OR IF YOU DEVELOP A FEVER.

WHEN USED AT THE RECOMMENDED DOSAGE FOR NO MORE THAN TWO DAYS, LOPERAMIDE AND OTHER ANTIDIARRHEAL MEDICATIONS RARELY CAUSE SIDE EFFECTS. BUT IF THE DIARRHEA DOES NOT DECREASE WITHIN ONE OR TWO DAYS, CHECK WITH YOUR DOCTOR.

MAGNESIUM

VITAL STATISTICS

GENERAL DESCRIPTION

Magnesium contributes to health in many ways. Along with calcium and phosphorus, it is a main ingredient of bone. A proper balance of calcium and magnesium is essential for healthy bones and teeth, reduces the risk of osteoporosis, and may alleviate existing osteoporosis. Calcium and magnesium also help regulate muscle activity; calcium stimulates contraction, magnesium induces relaxation. Magnesium is essential for metabolism and for building proteins. Adequate blood levels of magnesium protect the body from cardiovascular disease, heart arrhythmias, and possibly, stroke due to blood clotting in the brain.

The body's need for magnesium increases with stress or illness. Given as a supplement, magnesium may treat insomnia, muscle cramps, premenstrual syndrome, and cardiovascular problems including hypertension, angina due to coronary artery spasm, and pain and cramping due to insufficient blood flow to the legs. Studies indicate that giving magnesium immediately to a heart attack patient greatly increases the chance of survival.

The body processes magnesium efficiently; the kidneys conserve it as needed and excrete any excess amounts, so the incidences of both severe deficiency and toxicity are rare. These conditions are dangerous when they do occur, however.

Many over-the-counter antacids, laxatives, and analgesics contain magnesium, but these medications should not be used as magnesium supplements. A multinutrient supplement is a relatively safe way to augment your magnesium intake. Of the supplemental forms, magnesium citrate-malate is the easiest to absorb, while magnesium glycinate is the least likely to cause diarrhea at high doses.

RDA
Men: 350 mg
Women: 280 mg
Pregnant women: 320 mg

NATURAL SOURCES

On average, people get enough (or nearly enough) magnesium in their diet. Fish, green leafy vegetables, milk, nuts, seeds, and whole grains are good sources.

PRECAUTIONS

☠ WARNING

Take specific magnesium supplements only under a doctor's supervision. Magnesium toxicity can cause diarrhea, fatigue, muscle weakness, and in extreme cases, severely depressed heart rate and blood pressure, shallow breathing, loss of reflexes, coma, and even death. People who abuse laxatives or experience kidney failure are the most vulnerable to magnesium poisoning.

SPECIAL INFORMATION

Magnesium deficiency may cause nausea, vomiting, listlessness, muscle weakness, tremor, disorientation, and heart palpitations.

TARGET AILMENTS

Heart disease

Menstrual problems

Muscle cramps

SIDE EFFECTS
NONE EXPECTED

MAGNESIUM CARBONATE

VITAL STATISTICS

DRUG CLASS
Antacids

BRAND NAMES
Bayer Buffered Aspirin Tablets, Bufferin, Gaviscon (formula with aluminum hydroxide)

OTHER DRUGS IN THIS CLASS
aluminum hydroxide, calcium carbonate, magnesium hydroxide, sodium bicarbonate and citric acid

GENERAL DESCRIPTION
An active ingredient in some antacid medications, magnesium carbonate helps relieve symptoms of heartburn, sour stomach, acid indigestion, and upset stomach caused by diseases such as peptic ulcer, gastritis, esophagitis, and hiatal hernia. Magnesium carbonate is also used in combination with aspirin to increase the speed at which that drug dissolves, thereby reducing irritation in the gastrointestinal tract.

See Antacids for more information, including possible drug interactions and special information about this class of medications.

PRECAUTIONS

☠ WARNING
Except under medical supervision, do not take magnesium carbonate (or any antacid containing a magnesium compound) if you have impaired kidney function. Doing so could result in reduced blood pressure, nausea and vomiting, respiratory distress, and even coma.

TARGET AILMENTS

Upset stomach; heartburn; acid indigestion; sour stomach

Ulcers; gastritis; esophagitis

Pain (when used as a buffering ingredient with aspirin)

SIDE EFFECTS

NOT SERIOUS
- Mild diarrhea or mild constipation
- Increased thirst
- Unpleasant taste in mouth
- Stomach cramps; belching; flatulence
- Change in stool color (white or speckled)

CALL YOUR DOCTOR IF THESE PROBLEMS PERSIST.

SERIOUS
- Muscle pain or weakness
- Frequent or urgent urination
- Nausea; vomiting; dizziness; loss of appetite
- Nervousness or change in mood
- Fatigue
- Swollen ankles and feet
- Headache
- Bone pain

CONTACT YOUR DOCTOR IMMEDIATELY.

MAGNESIUM HYDROXIDE

VITAL STATISTICS

DRUG CLASS
Antacids

BRAND NAMES
Phillips' Milk of Magnesia, Rolaids, some types of Maalox and Mylanta

OTHER DRUGS IN THIS CLASS
aluminum hydroxide, calcium carbonate, magnesium carbonate, sodium bicarbonate and citric acid

GENERAL DESCRIPTION
Magnesium hydroxide is a magnesium-containing antacid drug used to relieve symptoms of upset and sour stomach, acid indigestion, heartburn, and ulcers. It is most effective when taken on an empty stomach. The most common side effect of magnesium hydroxide is a laxative action or diarrhea. See Antacids for information about possible drug interactions and additional special information.

PRECAUTIONS

SPECIAL INFORMATION
- Magnesium-containing antacids increase the risk of magnesium toxicity; do not take these drugs if you have kidney disease.
- Notify your doctor if you develop symptoms such as black, tarry stools or vomit the consistency of coffee grounds. These are indications of bleeding in the stomach or intestines.

TARGET AILMENTS

Upset stomach; heartburn; acid indigestion; sour stomach

Ulcers

SIDE EFFECTS

NOT SERIOUS
- Mild constipation
- Laxative effect or diarrhea
- Chalky taste in the mouth
- Stomach cramps; nausea or vomiting
- Belching
- Flatulence
- White specks in the stool

CALL YOUR DOCTOR IF THESE PROBLEMS PERSIST.

SERIOUS
- Swelling of the wrist, foot, or lower leg
- Bone pain
- Severe constipation
- Dizziness
- Mood changes
- Muscle pain, weakness, or twitching
- Nervousness or restlessness
- Slow breathing
- Irregular heartbeat
- Fatigue
- Pain upon urinating or frequent need to urinate
- Change in appetite

CONTACT YOUR DOCTOR IMMEDIATELY.

MELATONIN

VITAL STATISTICS

GENERAL DESCRIPTION

Melatonin is a hormone that occurs naturally in the body. It helps to regulate the body's daily biological rhythms. The hormone is released in cyclical patterns during each 24-hour period. The level of melatonin is determined by the amount of light present. During the day, very little melatonin is present in the body. But at night, the pineal gland synthesizes and releases the hormone into the bloodstream. Melatonin plays a role in determining the quality and length of sleep. Nighttime levels of the hormone decrease significantly in the elderly, who often have trouble getting to sleep and tend to sleep for fewer hours.

Melatonin may help protect the immune system by minimizing the potentially damaging effects of high amounts of steroid hormones called corticosteroids. Chronic high levels of corticosteroids have been linked with glucose intolerance, impaired immune function, and clogged arteries—all factors associated with aging. Melatonin's effect on corticosteroids is one reason melatonin has been said to be able to combat aging. Animal research suggests the hormone also plays a role in suppressing the growth of certain cancer tumors.

Melatonin supplements were introduced in the U.S. market in the early 1990s. It is best known as a sleeping aid. Small amounts of the supplement taken after airplane flights that cross several time zones help alleviate jet lag. The supplements can also be effective in inducing sleep in people with insomnia, particularly the elderly, and in shift workers.

Proponents of melatonin claim the supplements boost the immune system, slow the aging process, and fight cancer, although these effects have not been proved in studies on human beings.

PREPARATIONS

In the United States, melatonin is sold as a dietary supplement in tablet and capsule form.

PRECAUTIONS

☠ WARNING

Do not take melatonin if you are pregnant.

SPECIAL INFORMATION

Little is known about the effects of taking melatonin on a long-term basis. Because it is a potent hormone, some experts argue it should be regulated as a drug, as it is in Canada and Germany, and not as a dietary supplement, as it is in the United States. Animal research suggests melatonin can be harmful for people with autoimmune diseases, such as multiple sclerosis, or those with collagen-induced arthritis.

TARGET AILMENTS

Jet lag; insomnia; stress

Seasonal affective disorder (SAD)

Cancer (adjunct therapy)

SIDE EFFECTS

- Headache; rash; upset stomach
- Disruption of normal circadian rhythm

DISCONTINUE USE AND CALL YOUR DOCTOR.

METHYL SALICYLATE

VITAL STATISTICS

DRUG CLASS
Analgesics [Topical Analgesics]

BRAND NAME
Ben-Gay

OTHER DRUGS IN THIS CLASS
acetaminophen, aspirin, nonsteroidal anti-in-flammatory drugs (NSAIDs), opioid analgesics

GENERAL DESCRIPTION
Obtained from the leaves and bark of plants in the *Gaultheria,* birch, and poplar families, or produced synthetically, methyl salicylate is used as a topical medicine for relieving pain in muscles and joints. Sometimes called wintergreen oil, the substance works as a counter-irritant; it stimulates skin receptors, providing temporary relief from aches and pains.

Methyl salicylate is available in a variety of gels, liniments, lotions, and ointments, usually in combination with menthol or camphor. The concentration of methyl salicylate in these products varies from 10 to 60 percent. Poisonous if ingested, methyl salicylate is relatively safe for external use.

PRECAUTIONS

SPECIAL INFORMATION
- Heat and humidity increase the absorption of methyl salicylate through the skin, thus increasing the risk of salicylate toxicity. Do not exercise vigorously in hot, humid weather after application or use a heating pad immediately after application.
- To reduce risk of irritation, avoid contact with eyes; mucous membranes; or broken, irritated skin.

TARGET AILMENTS

Minor muscle and joint aches and pains from arthritis, sprains, strains, and bruises (use only if skin is intact)

SIDE EFFECTS

NOT SERIOUS
- Local skin redness or irritation

DISCONTINUE USE AND CONTACT YOUR DOCTOR IF THESE EFFECTS BECOME TROUBLESOME.

SERIOUS
- Salicylate toxicity (dizziness, ringing in ears, nausea, vomiting), a rare condition caused by absorption through the skin into the blood

DISCONTINUE USE AND CONTACT YOUR DOCTOR.

R✕ MICONAZOLE

VITAL STATISTICS

DRUG CLASS
Antifungal Drugs

BRAND NAMES
Rx: Monistat-Derm, Monistat Dual-Pak, Monistat 3 Vaginal Suppositories
OTC: Monistat 7

OTHER DRUGS IN THIS CLASS
Rx: clotrimazole, fluconazole, ketoconazole, terconazole
OTC: clotrimazole, tolnaftate, undecylenate

GENERAL DESCRIPTION
Miconazole, available in topical and vaginal preparations, is used to treat a variety of fungal infections. See Antifungal Drugs for more information. For information about other medications commonly used to treat vaginal yeast infections, see Vaginal Antifungal Drugs.

PRECAUTIONS

SPECIAL INFORMATION
- Topical creams, lotions, and powders are applied directly to the skin to combat the fungi that cause body ringworm, jock itch, and athlete's foot. They can be used twice a day for up to one month.
- Vaginal creams and suppositories are inserted directly into the vagina, usually at bedtime, for a period of three to seven days.

POSSIBLE INTERACTIONS
No interactions are expected with most topical and vaginal forms of antifungal drugs.

TARGET AILMENTS

Yeast infections (candidiasis) of the vulva and vagina, mouth, skin, hands, and internal organs

Ringworm (tinea) of the body, scalp, nails, hands, feet (athlete's foot), and groin (jock itch)

Tinea versicolor, a ringworm infection that produces white-brown patches on the skin

Fungal skin infections (topical)

SIDE EFFECTS

NOT SERIOUS
- Mild skin irritation in the infected area
- Headache; drowsiness
- Dizziness; nausea; vomiting
- Stomach pain
- Constipation or diarrhea

CALL YOUR DOCTOR IF THESE EFFECTS PERSIST.

SERIOUS
- Allergic skin reactions, such as a rash or hives (topical preparations)
- Redness, stinging, burning, or itching of the genitals; abdominal cramps or menstrual irregularities; or itching and burning of a sexual partner's penis (vaginal preparations)

CALL YOUR DOCTOR AT ONCE.

MILK THISTLE

LATIN NAME
Silybum marianum

VITAL STATISTICS

GENERAL DESCRIPTION

Milk thistle, a plant that reaches five feet in height and thrives both in the wild and in the garden, is used by herbalists to treat such liver disorders as cirrhosis and hepatitis. The active ingredient, silymarin, is found in the seeds. It is believed that silymarin prompts the manufacture of new, healthy liver cells without encouraging the growth of any malignant liver tissue that may be present. Silymarin, it is thought, also serves as an antioxidant, protecting liver cells from damage by free radicals, which are harmful by-products of many bodily processes, including cellular metabolism. The use of silymarin by healthy people can increase by as much as one-third the liver's content of glutathione, a key substance in detoxifying many potentially damaging hormones, chemicals, and drugs.

Extracts of silymarin appear to neutralize toxins from the death cup mushroom, which can inflict lethal injury on the liver. Milk thistle is also believed to ease outbreaks of psoriasis, since these may worsen when the liver fails to neutralize certain toxins that circulate in the bloodstream.

PREPARATIONS

Over the counter:
Available in dried bulk, capsules, and extract.

At home:
TEA: Steep covered 1 tsp freshly ground seeds in 1 cup boiling water for 10 to 15 minutes; drink three times daily. As an alternative to tea, eat 1 tsp freshly ground seeds. Milk thistle extract may be more effective than teas, since silymarin is only slightly soluble in water. See a herbalist for further information. Consult a qualified practitioner for the dosage appropriate for your specific condition.

TARGET AILMENTS

Liver problems, including cirrhosis and hepatitis

Inflammation of the gallbladder duct

Poisoning from ingestion of the death cup mushroom

Psoriasis

SIDE EFFECTS

NOT SERIOUS

BECAUSE TAKING MILK THISTLE INCREASES BILE SECRETION, YOU MAY DEVELOP LOOSE STOOLS.

PRECAUTIONS

☠ WARNING

If you think that you have a liver disorder, seek medical advice.

SPECIAL INFORMATION

Use of this herb by children for more than seven to 10 days should be done in conjunction with a healthcare practitioner.

POSSIBLE INTERACTIONS

Combining milk thistle with other herbs may necessitate a lower dosage.

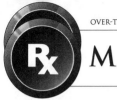

MINOXIDIL

VITAL STATISTICS

DRUG CLASS
Hair Growth Stimulants

BRAND NAME
Rogaine

GENERAL DESCRIPTION
As a topical solution, minoxidil is used to treat baldness in both men and women. Under proper conditions, preparations containing 2 percent minoxidil may stimulate the growth of new hair on the scalp. These stimulating effects are more noticeable in younger people and in those with early male-pattern baldness. Although the exact mechanism of action is not established, researchers believe that minoxidil increases blood flow near the skin's surface, resulting in the stimulation of hair follicle cells. However, once treatment is stopped, new hair will fall out, which is why many people choose to use minoxidil indefinitely. Minoxidil preparations can also be used as supportive therapy in hair transplants.

Minoxidil was originally designed as an oral antihypertensive drug; as such, misuse or absorption of the drug into your system can have serious side effects. Those who use minoxidil as a topical hair growth stimulant should not have any heart problems, and they must have healthy scalps. When this drug is used as an oral antihypertensive, 4 out of 5 patients experience a side effect of thicker, longer, and darker body hair after three to six weeks.

PRECAUTIONS

☠ WARNING
Do not take this medication if you have an adrenaline-producing tumor (pheochromocytoma).

SPECIAL INFORMATION
- Minoxidil topical preparations may be absorbed into your system after prolonged use. Possible side effects of systemic absorption include fast heartbeat, edema, and low blood pressure.
- Use this drug with caution if you have cardiovascular disease or hypertension. Talk with your doctor about the risks involved.
- The actual dosage and use of topical preparations should be individualized. In most cases, a thin application twice daily to the entire scalp will suffice. Follow package and doctor's instructions carefully.
- Skin abrasions or irritations such as psoriasis, sunburn, and flaking skin may worsen with use of topical minoxidil.
- Oral minoxidil crosses the placenta. Women should discontinue use of minoxidil at least one month before birth-control measures are discontinued. Pregnant women or nursing mothers should discuss the risks of using minoxidil with their doctor.

CONTINUED

MINOXIDIL

POSSIBLE INTERACTIONS

Although no possible interactions are reported for the topical preparation, drug interactions are possible with other antihypertensive agents if systemic absorption occurs. Anyone taking antihypertensive drugs should be aware of the risks.

Oral minoxidil (concurrent use): toxicity may occur.

Topical adrenocorticoids, retinoids, and petrolatum products: may cause undesirable absorption of minoxidil.

TARGET AILMENTS

Baldness (alopecia)

Female androgenic baldness

Early male-pattern baldness (androgenic alopecia)

SIDE EFFECTS

NOT SERIOUS

- Allergic reaction, such as burning, itchy scalp, flaking, or reddening skin
- Increased baldness
- Dermatitis
- Headache; dizziness
- Sexual dysfunction
- Vision problems
- Increased hair growth in other areas
- Eczema; loss of hair; dry skin

CALL YOUR DOCTOR IF THESE EFFECTS PERSIST OR BECOME BOTHERSOME.

SERIOUS

- Chest pain; dizziness or faintness; fast, irregular heartbeat; hypotension; swelling in hands or feet from water retention; or vasodilation (signs of systemic absorption)
- Burning scalp; skin rash; unusual swelling or tingling in face, hands, feet; headache, flushing; rapid weight gain (rare)

DISCONTINUE USE AND SEEK EMERGENCY TREATMENT.

NEOMYCIN

VITAL STATISTICS

DRUG CLASS
Antibiotics [Topical Antibiotics]

BRAND NAME
Neosporin

OTHER DRUGS IN THIS SUBCLASS
Rx: chlorhexidine (for gums); mupirocin (for skin); combination of neomycin, polymyxin B, and hydrocortisone (antibiotic-corticosteroid for ears or eyes)
OTC: bacitracin, polymyxin B

GENERAL DESCRIPTION
Neomycin is an aminoglycoside, an antibiotic with a broad spectrum of activity and effectiveness. In oral forms the drug can be used to treat gastrointestinal infections, although it is rarely given orally because of the high risk of kidney and hearing damage. Neomycin is available over the counter as a topical ointment by itself, or in combination with polymyxin B and bacitracin. This combination is used on the skin to prevent infections in minor cuts, scrapes, and burns.

By prescription, neomycin comes in combination with polymyxin B and hydrocortisone for a combined antibiotic and corticosteroid treatment for external ear infections. Other forms of these three drugs are used to treat bacterial infections of the eye and skin. For more information, see Topical Antibiotics.

PRECAUTIONS

SPECIAL INFORMATION
- Check with your doctor if you notice no improvement after using these medications for two or three days.
- The use of topical antibiotics increases the risk of kidney damage or hearing loss in people with impaired kidney function who are already taking nephrotoxic medicines.
- If you are pregnant or nursing, check with your doctor before using.

POSSIBLE INTERACTIONS
Other aminoglycosides: possible hypersensitivity reaction and toxicity leading to permanent deafness.

TARGET AILMENTS
Minor cuts, scrapes, and burns (neomycin alone, or in combination with bacitracin and polymyxin B, to prevent bacterial infection)

External ear canal infections (neomycin, polymyxin B, and hydrocortisone in combination)

SIDE EFFECTS

SERIOUS
- Allergic reaction such as itching, stinging, rash, redness, or swelling at the application site
- Kidney damage or hearing loss (due to extensive systemic absorption of neomycin via application over large areas of the body or through prolonged use)

CALL YOUR DOCTOR IMMEDIATELY.

NIACIN (VITAMIN B3)

VITAL STATISTICS

OTHER NAME
vitamin B_3

GENERAL DESCRIPTION
Niacin contributes to more than 50 vital bodily processes. Among other things, it helps convert food into energy; build red blood cells; synthesize hormones, fatty acids, and steroids; maintain skin, nerves, and blood vessels; support the gastrointestinal tract; stabilize mental health; and detoxify certain drugs and chemicals in the body. In addition, it helps insulin regulate blood sugar levels. Niacin is also a powerful drug, capable of lowering blood cholesterol and triglycerides, dilating blood vessels to improve circulation, and alleviating depression, insomnia, and hyperactivity.

Extreme deficiency of niacin results in pellagra, characterized by diarrhea, dermatitis, and mental illness. Pellagra was common until the discovery that niacin was a cure; the disease is now virtually nonexistent in the United States thanks to niacin-enriched flour and other foods. Multivitamin supplements can raise niacin levels safely.

RDA
Men: 19 mg
Women: 15 mg
Pregnant women: 17 mg

NATURAL SOURCES
Niacin-rich foods include liver, poultry, lean meats, fish, nuts, peanut butter, and enriched flour. If you get enough protein, you are probably receiving adequate niacin as well. If adequate vitamin B_6 is present, the body can also produce niacin from the amino acid tryptophan, found in milk, eggs, and cheese.

PRECAUTIONS

☠ WARNING
Niacin is toxic in high amounts, so large doses should be taken only under a doctor's supervision. Nausea is the first symptom, which often prevents further intake; continued overuse may cause a rash, itchy skin, and liver damage.

SPECIAL INFORMATION
- Signs of niacin deficiency include indigestion; diarrhea; muscle weakness; loss of appetite; dermatitis that is worsened by exposure to sunlight; mouth sores; a red, inflamed tongue; headaches; irritability; anxiety; and depression.
- Pregnant or breast-feeding women, the elderly, alcoholics, and people with hyperthyroidism are the most likely to be niacin deficient.

TARGET AILMENTS
Depression

High cholesterol

SIDE EFFECTS
NONE EXPECTED

NONSTEROIDAL ANTI-INFLAMMATORY DRUGS (NSAIDs)

VITAL STATISTICS

GENERIC NAMES
Rx: diclofenac, etodolac, flurbiprofen, ibuprofen, ketoprofen, ketorolac, nabumetone, naproxen, oxaprozin
OTC: ibuprofen, ketoprofen, naproxen

GENERAL DESCRIPTION
NSAIDs are nonnarcotic analgesic drugs that reduce inflammation, especially from arthritis. These drugs are used by people who cannot tolerate aspirin, or when aspirin or acetaminophen is not effective. In addition to reducing inflammation, NSAIDs relieve pain. Some are indicated for reducing fever.

TARGET AILMENTS

Inflammation, especially related to osteoarthritis and rheumatoid arthritis

Pain, especially from inflammation, dental and other surgeries, menstruation, or migraines

Fever

PRECAUTIONS

SPECIAL INFORMATION
- If NSAIDs upset your stomach, take them with food or milk.
- Do not use NSAIDs if you are allergic to them or to aspirin. NSAIDs may cause bronchoconstriction or anaphylaxis in aspirin-sensitive asthmatics.
- Avoid these drugs or consult your doctor before using them if you have asthma, peptic ulcer, enteritis (intestinal inflammation), high blood pressure, bleeding problems, epilepsy, Parkinson's disease, or impaired liver or kidney function.
- Do not take more than the recommended dose and seek emergency help in case of overdose. Possible symptoms of overdose include drowsiness, increased sweating, rapid heartbeat, abdominal pain, vomiting, nausea, gastrointestinal bleeding, and disorientation.
- NSAIDs are not recommended for pregnant women, especially during the last trimester, or for nursing mothers.

POSSIBLE INTERACTIONS
Because NSAIDs interact with many substances, check with your doctor or pharmacist before taking in combination with other drugs. NSAIDs can affect liver and kidney function, thereby increasing the toxicity of other drugs. Some or all NSAIDs can interact with the following drugs:
Acetaminophen: increased risk of adverse liver or kidney effect.
Alcohol: possible bleeding and ulcers.
Antacids: decreased NSAID effect.
Anticoagulant drugs: increased anticoagulant effect, possible bleeding.

CONTINUED

NONSTEROIDAL ANTI-INFLAMMATORY DRUGS (NSAIDs)

Anticonvulsant drugs (phenytoin): increased action of phenytoin.

Antidiabetic drugs and insulin: increased hypoglycemic effect; with diclofenac, either increased or decreased hypoglycemic effect.

Antipsychotic drugs (such as chlorpromazine and clozapine): with nabumetone, decreased effects of these drugs.

Aspirin: increased risk of stomach problems.

Benzodiazepines (such as chlordiazepoxide, diazepam, and oxazepam): with nabumetone, decreased effects of these drugs.

Beta-adrenergic blockers: decreased antihypertensive effect.

Cimetidine: may increase or decrease the effect of the NSAID.

Colchicine: possibility of bleeding and ulcers when combined with certain NSAIDs.

Corticosteroids: possible bleeding and ulcers. Don't combine unless directed to do so by your doctor.

Cyclosporine: increased risk of kidney damage.

Diuretics: reduced diuretic effect.

Methotrexate: increased toxicity of methotrexate; possibly fatal poisoning.

Probenecid: increased NSAID effect, possible NSAID toxicity.

Sulfonamides: possible sulfonamide toxicity.

Tricyclic antidepressants (such as amitriptyline): with nabumetone, decreased effects of these drugs.

Verapamil: increased toxicity.

SIDE EFFECTS

NOT SERIOUS

- Dizziness
- Drowsiness
- Headache
- Abdominal pain or cramps
- Constipation
- Diarrhea; heartburn
- Nausea

CONSULT YOUR DOCTOR IF THESE SYMPTOMS PERSIST.

SERIOUS

- Hives, rash, intense itching, and trouble breathing (anaphylactic reaction)

SEEK EMERGENCY HELP.

- Chest pain or irregular heartbeat
- Diminished hearing or ringing in the ears
- Trouble breathing
- Fluid retention
- Black or tarry stools
- Blood in urine
- Photosensitivity
- Jaundice (indicated by bleeding, bruising, tiredness, tenderness in upper abdomen, and yellow eyes or skin)
- Gastrointestinal ulceration, bleeding, and perforation of stomach

DISCONTINUE USE AND CALL YOUR DOCTOR IMMEDIATELY IF YOU NOTICE ANY OF THESE SYMPTOMS.

OMEGA-3 FATTY ACIDS

GENERAL DESCRIPTION

Omega-3 fatty acids have earned a wide reputation for preventing heart disease. They are linked to low incidences of heart disease in world populations that eat large amounts of fatty fish. These fatty acids help lower blood levels of LDL, the harmful type of cholesterol that can lead to atherosclerosis. Omega-3 fatty acids also contribute to functions in the body that help thin the blood and decrease plaque along artery walls, improving blood circulation.

Omega-3 fatty acids may relieve inflammation associated with colitis or arthritis, and skin problems such as skin cancer or psoriasis. Purported to have overall health benefits, omega-3 fatty acids are sometimes recommended to treat kidney problems, multiple sclerosis, and cancer, among other ailments.

NATURAL SOURCES

cold-water fish, including tuna, salmon, mackerel, and sardines; walnuts; flaxseed oil; canola oil

PREPARATIONS

Available in flaxseed, flaxseed oil, and gel capsules.

TARGET AILMENTS

Heart disease; high cholesterol; arthritis; colitis; psoriasis; atopic dermatitis (eczema); lupus; multiple sclerosis; cancer

PRECAUTIONS

☠ WARNING

Avoid concentrated supplements unless recommended by your doctor.

Omega-3 fatty acids may slow blood clotting. Do not take these supplements if you have a blood-clotting disorder.

SPECIAL INFORMATION

- No standard recommended dosage has been determined. Consult your doctor for advice on adding omega-3 fatty acids to your diet. Most doctors recommend eating fish rather than taking supplements.
- If you are pregnant or breast-feeding, consult your doctor before taking supplements.
- With excessive amounts, unusual bleeding may result.
- Omega-3 fatty acid supplements may raise blood levels of HDL, the good kind of cholesterol, causing an increase in overall blood cholesterol levels.

POSSIBLE INTERACTIONS

Anticoagulant medications, including aspirin: may increase anticoagulant effect. Consult your doctor before taking omega-3 fatty acid supplements.

SIDE EFFECTS

NOT SERIOUS
- Unusual tiredness (anemia)

CALL YOUR DOCTOR.

OXYMETAZOLINE

VITAL STATISTICS

DRUG CLASS
Decongestants

BRAND NAMES
Afrin, Neo-Synephrine Maximum Strength

OTHER DRUGS IN THIS CLASS
Rx: phenylpropanolamine
OTC: phenylephrine, phenylpropanolamine, pseudoephedrine

GENERAL DESCRIPTION
Used as an active ingredient in over-the-counter nose sprays, oxymetazoline relieves nasal congestion caused by colds, allergies, or sinusitis by constricting blood vessels in nasal passages. Its best use is as a short-term (over several days) decongestant. While short-term use as directed on the label usually produces minimal side effects, long-term use or overuse may result in rebound congestion or absorption into the bloodstream, producing central nervous system effects similar to those of oral decongestants (dizziness, headache, insomnia, nervousness, high blood pressure, heart-rhythm problems). For more information, see Decongestants.

TARGET AILMENTS

Congestion of the nose and sinuses caused by allergy or upper respiratory infection

PRECAUTIONS

SPECIAL INFORMATION
Check with your doctor before taking this drug if you have cardiovascular disease (including angina, coronary artery disease, and hypertension), hyperthyroidism (overactive thyroid), diabetes, prostate enlargement, or glaucoma. Oxymetazoline may exacerbate these conditions.

POSSIBLE INTERACTIONS
Tricyclic antidepressants (such as amitriptyline): increased serious central nervous system side effects if oxymetazoline is absorbed into the bloodstream.

SIDE EFFECTS

NOT SERIOUS
- Sneezing
- Burning, stinging, or dryness of nose

  CONSULT YOUR DOCTOR IF SYMPTOMS CONTINUE OR ARE BOTHERSOME.

SERIOUS
- Severe headache; trembling
- Nervousness or restlessness
- Insomnia
- Pounding or irregular heartbeat
- High blood pressure
- Rebound congestion

CALL YOUR DOCTOR RIGHT AWAY.

PEPPERMINT

LATIN NAME
Mentha x piperita

VITAL STATISTICS

GENERAL DESCRIPTION

Peppermint plants have long, serrated leaves and a familiar, minty aroma. This pleasant-tasting herb has been used as a remedy for indigestion since the era of ancient Egypt. Menthol, the principal active ingredient of peppermint, stimulates the stomach lining, thereby reducing the amount of time food spends in the stomach. It also relaxes the muscles of the digestive system. Peppermint can be grown easily from root cuttings; but if it is not confined, it tends to spread rapidly.

PREPARATIONS

Over the counter:
Peppermint is available as commercial tea, tinctures, and fresh or dried leaves and flowers.

At home:
TEA: Drink commercial brands, or steep covered 1 to 2 heaping tsp dried herb per cup of boiling water for 10 minutes. Drink up to 3 cups a day.
BATH: Fill a cloth bag with several handfuls of dried or fresh herb and let hot water run over it.
COMBINATIONS: For colds and flu, peppermint may be used as a tea or tincture with boneset, elder flower, and yarrow.
Consult a qualified practitioner for the dosage appropriate for you and the specific condition being treated.

SIDE EFFECTS
NONE EXPECTED

PRECAUTIONS

☠ WARNING

Do not ingest pure menthol or pure peppermint oil; these substances are extremely toxic. Pure peppermint oil may cause cardiac arrhythmias, and pure menthol can be fatal in a dose as small as a teaspoon.

Give only very dilute preparations to children younger than two years old and only under the supervision of a doctor or herbalist.

Pregnant women with morning sickness should use a dilute tea rather than a more potent infusion. Peppermint should not be used by women who have a history of miscarriage.

POSSIBLE INTERACTIONS

Combining peppermint with other herbs may necessitate a lower dosage.

TARGET AILMENTS

Take internally for:

Cramps (including menstrual); stomach pain

Gas; nausea associated with migraine headaches

Morning sickness; travel sickness

Insomnia; anxiety

Fever; colds; flu

Apply tea externally for:

Itching; inflammation

PERMETHRIN

VITAL STATISTICS

DRUG CLASS
Antilouse Drugs

BRAND NAMES
Nix Creme Rinse, Elimite

GENERAL DESCRIPTION
Permethrin is the active component in most over-the-counter preparations for the topical treatment of head lice. This drug kills both living insects, by attacking their nervous systems and paralyzing them, and their tiny white eggs (nits) attached to human hairs. Permethrin does not have the potent side effects of other, more toxic antilouse drugs.

Permethrin is found in medicated shampoos and hair-rinse products, and also in a 5 percent cream formula for treating scabies (caused by mites). Most preparations work well with a single application, but a second application five to seven days after the first may sometimes be necessary. Protective residues of the product remain in the hair for 10 to 14 days.

Most permethrin preparations can effectively treat three different kinds of lice infestations—head, pubic, and body lice. However, a 1 percent permethrin creme-rinse product that protects the head from head lice reinfestation for a full 14 days is not approved by the FDA as safe and effective for treating pubic lice or body lice.

PRECAUTIONS

☠ WARNING
Susceptible individuals may experience breathing difficulty or an asthmatic reaction when using any form of this product.

SPECIAL INFORMATION
- Individuals sensitive to ragweed, chrysanthemums, pyrethrins, or veterinary insecticides containing permethrin are likely to be sensitive to all permethrin products.
- This is a topical medication. It should not be taken orally or internally. If swallowed, immediately call your doctor and/or a poison control center.
- Avoid getting this medication near or in the eyes. If you accidentally get permethrin in your eyes, flush them thoroughly with water.
- Permethrin is not recommended for children under two years of age.
- A second application is necessary if live lice are observed seven days after the first application.

PERMETHRIN

- Nursing mothers should either not use permethrin or consider temporarily discontinuing breast-feeding while using it.
- Directions for the use of these products must be followed carefully to ensure total disinfection. Careful attention must be paid to the disinfection of all clothing, headgear, bedding, and personal belongings where insects can hide.

TARGET AILMENTS

Head, pubic, and body lice

Scabies (caused by mites)

SIDE EFFECTS

NOT SERIOUS

- Itching, burning, stinging, tingling skin
- Swelling; rash
- Numbness; discomfort
- Possible asthmatic reactions
- Temporary increased itching, redness, stinging, or swelling of the scalp (accompanies lice infestations)

CALL YOUR DOCTOR IF THESE EFFECTS PERSIST OR BECOME BOTHERSOME.

PHENOL

VITAL STATISTICS

DRUG CLASS
Antiseptics

BRAND NAMES
Anbesol, Chloraseptic

GENERAL DESCRIPTION
Phenol was discovered in 1834 as a component of coal tar (hence its other name, carbolic acid). Used alone, phenol is extremely toxic and potentially fatal, so this antiseptic is used only in small amounts and in combination with other chemicals. These preparations are used to inhibit the growth of bacteria and to reduce the chance of infection in minor scrapes, cuts, and burns. Sometimes phenol is included in preparations used to treat poison ivy rashes and insect bites, or to relieve the pain associated with toothaches, teething, fever blisters, and other soreness of the gums, mouth, and throat. Combined with certain other drugs, such as benzocaine, phenol has an analgesic or local anesthetic effect, which makes it useful in temporarily reducing pain and itching when applied directly on the skin.

TARGET AILMENTS

Minor cuts, scrapes, and burns

Local infections

Pain and soreness of gums and mouth

Pain and itching due to insect bites or poison ivy

SIDE EFFECTS

NOT SERIOUS

WHEN USED ACCORDING TO PACKAGE LABEL INSTRUCTIONS, PRODUCTS CONTAINING PHENOL ARE CONSIDERED SAFE AND EFFECTIVE AND VERY RARELY PRODUCE SIDE EFFECTS.

SERIOUS

- Irritation
- Pain
- Redness
- Rash
- Swelling
- Fever

DISCONTINUE USE AND CONTACT YOUR DOCTOR IMMEDIATELY.

PHENOL

☠ WARNING

Overuse or overapplication of this drug can lead to serious, potentially life-threatening side effects.

SPECIAL INFORMATION

- Although some preparations containing phenol are specially formulated for use in the mouth or throat, this drug is potentially fatal if swallowed in large enough amounts. Keep this drug away from children.
- Do not use phenol if you are allergic to local anesthetics containing benzocaine.
- Do not use this drug near the eyes.
- Do not use on children under age two or for diaper rash, as this medication is easily absorbed into the skin.
- Do not apply topical preparations over large areas of skin, and never cover the treated area with a bandage or dressing.
- Do not use for longer than seven days; if the irritation has not improved within that period, see your doctor or dentist.
- If you are pregnant or nursing, check with your doctor before using this drug.
- To treat a teething baby, use only the recommended amount. Do not overdose.
- If you have an infection or many sores in your mouth, check with your doctor or dentist before using oral preparations containing phenol.

POSSIBLE INTERACTIONS

Phenol preparations have not been shown to interact with any specific drugs. However, before using these medications, be sure to inform your doctor, dentist, or pharmacist of any other prescription or nonprescription drug you are taking.

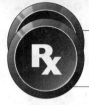

PHENYLPROPANOLAMINE

VITAL STATISTICS

DRUG CLASS
Decongestants

BRAND NAMES
Rx: Entex LA
OTC: Alka-Seltzer Plus, Comtrex Liqui-Gel, Dexatrim (diet aid), Dimetapp (for adults and children), Naldecon-DX, Robitussin-CF, Tavist-D, Triaminic DM Syrup, Triaminic Expectorant, Triaminicol Multi-Symptom Relief, Triaminic Syrup, Tylenol Cold (effervescent formula)

OTHER DRUGS IN THIS CLASS
OTC: oxymetazoline, phenylephrine, pseudoephedrine

GENERAL DESCRIPTION
A nasal decongestant sometimes used as an appetite suppressant, phenylpropanolamine is widely used in over-the-counter cold and allergy products. This medication is banned for use during athletic competitions. For more information, see Decongestants.

PRECAUTIONS

SPECIAL INFORMATION
- In rare cases, phenylpropanolamine has been associated with serious cardiovascular, central nervous system, and psychological effects such as stroke, irregular heart rhythms, high blood pressure, hallucinations, and seizures. These effects may be more likely in individuals who take high dosages or who have an underlying cardiovascular or psychological illness.
- Check with your doctor before taking this drug if you have cardiovascular disease (including angina, coronary artery disease, and hypertension), hyperthyroidism (overactive thyroid), diabetes, or glaucoma. Phenylpropanolamine may exacerbate these conditions.

TARGET AILMENTS
Congestion of the nose and sinuses

Bronchial asthma

Obesity (used as an appetite suppressant)

Urinary incontinence

PHENYLPROPANOLAMINE

POSSIBLE INTERACTIONS

Anticoagulant (blood-thinning) drugs: decreased anticoagulant effect.

Beta blockers: phenylpropanolamine can lessen the effectiveness of beta blockers, causing hypertension.

Digitalis preparations: possible heart-rhythm problems.

High blood pressure drugs containing rauwolfia: decreased effectiveness of phenylpropanolamine.

Monoamine oxidase (MAO) inhibitors: increased stimulant action of phenylpropanolamine, causing effects such as hypertension and heart-rhythm problems.

Stimulants (such as other decongestants, amphetamines, caffeine): increased stimulant effects, leading to excessive nervousness, insomnia, irregular heart rhythm, or seizures.

Tricyclic antidepressants (such as amitriptyline): increased action of phenylpropanolamine, making serious central nervous system side effects more likely.

SIDE EFFECTS

NOT SERIOUS

- Mild nervousness
- Restlessness
- Insomnia
- Dizziness
- Lightheadedness
- Nausea
- Dryness of mouth or nose
- Rebound congestion

CALL YOUR DOCTOR IF THESE EFFECTS PERSIST OR BECOME BOTHERSOME.

SERIOUS

- Stroke
- Irregular heart rhythms
- High blood pressure
- Hallucinations
- Seizures

CALL YOUR DOCTOR IMMEDIATELY.

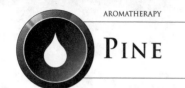

PINE

LATIN NAME
Pinus sylvestris

VITAL STATISTICS

GENERAL DESCRIPTION

The needles of the fragrant Scotch pine are used to produce pine oil, a safe, useful, and therapeutic oil said to have expectorant and decongestant properties. The oil is colorless to pale yellow, with a strong balsamic and camphoric aroma. It is used to treat pulmonary problems and the flu as well as other viral infections.

The Scotch pine is native to Eurasia and is most widespread in western and northern Europe and in Russia. The trees can grow up to 120 feet high. In earlier seafaring days, the trunks were prized as masts for sailing ships. Native Americans stuffed mattresses with the needles to repel fleas and lice. Today the Scotch pine, with its long, stiff needle pairs, is a favorite for decorating at Christmas.

PREPARATIONS

The oil can either be applied externally or inhaled to relieve respiratory problems or calm the mind. For a steam inhalation, place 6 drops in a bowl of boiling water. Lean over the bowl, drape a towel over your head and the bowl, and inhale for up to 5 minutes.

Add 10 to 15 drops to a warm bath to ease circulatory problems, swelling from arthritis and rheumatism, premenstrual syndrome, and anxious or depressed states of mind. Pine oil is also effective at countering urinary tract problems by using it in a sitz bath or applying it to the skin. For a massage oil, mix 10 to 15 drops in vegetable or nut oil or aloe gel. (Skin applications can be used for all target ailments.)

If the quality of the oil is suspect, a tea made from steeping pine needles in boiling water may substitute for pine oil.

PRECAUTIONS

SPECIAL INFORMATION

Buy only from a reputable source. Pine oil is easily adulterated with turpentine, which compromises its effectiveness.

TARGET AILMENTS

Anxiety; depression

Nervous tension

Skin disorders

Arthritis; rheumatism

Cystitis and other urinary problems

Bronchitis; sinus problems

Coughs; viral infections, including the flu

Pneumonia

SIDE EFFECTS

NOT SERIOUS

PINE CAN IRRITATE THE SKIN. AVOID USING THIS OIL IF YOU HAVE SENSITIVE SKIN.

POTASSIUM

VITAL STATISTICS

GENERAL DESCRIPTION

Potassium is the third most abundant mineral in the body, after calcium and phosphorus. It works closely with sodium and chloride to maintain fluid distribution and pH balance and to augment nerve-impulse transmission, muscle contraction, and regulation of heartbeat and blood pressure. Potassium is also required for protein synthesis, carbohydrate metabolism, and insulin secretion by the pancreas. Studies suggest that people who regularly eat potassium-rich foods are less likely to develop atherosclerosis, heart disease, and high blood pressure, or to die of a stroke.

Many Americans may get only marginal amounts of potassium, but supplements, such as potassium aspartate, are best taken only under a doctor's guidance.

Marginal potassium deficiency causes no symptoms but may increase the risk of developing high blood pressure or aggravate existing heart disease. More severe deficiency can result in constipation, muscle cramps and muscle weakness, poor reflexes, poor concentration, heart arrhythmias, and, rarely, death due to heart failure. Acute potassium toxicity may have similar effects, including possible heart failure. However, acute toxicity is rarely linked to diet and tends to occur only in the event of kidney failure.

EMDR
Adults: 2,000 mg

NATURAL SOURCES

Dietary sources include lean meats, raw vegetables, fruits (especially citrus fruits, bananas, and avocados), potatoes, and dandelion greens.

PRECAUTIONS

☠ WARNING

Consult a doctor before taking potassium supplements.

People with kidney disease should never take potassium supplements.

TARGET AILMENTS

Heart disease

High blood pressure

SIDE EFFECTS
NONE EXPECTED

PRAMOXINE

VITAL STATISTICS

DRUG CLASS
Anesthetics

BRAND NAMES
Caladryl, Fleet Hemorrhoidal Preparation, Anusol

OTHER DRUGS IN THIS CLASS
benzocaine, dyclonine

GENERAL DESCRIPTION
Pramoxine is a local anesthetic used topically for the temporary relief of pain, itching, and inflammation associated with minor skin disorders. It works by blocking nerve impulses to the brain. The drug is considered safe and effective for use by adults and children over the age of two, although it is not recommended for treatment of diaper rash. Pramoxine is chemically unrelated to other anesthetics, reducing the likelihood of cross-sensitivity reactions in people who are allergic to other local anesthetics. Drug interactions are uncommon, and it seldom causes serious side effects. See Anesthetics for additional information.

PRECAUTIONS

SPECIAL INFORMATION
- Pramoxine is for external use only. Avoid applying it over large areas, to open wounds, where there may be a risk of infection, or to broken skin. Keep this product away from the eyes, ears, or mouth.
- If the condition worsens, the problem area becomes infected, bleeding occurs, or symptoms persist for more than seven days, discontinue use and consult a physician.
- Before using this drug, seek the advice of your doctor if you are pregnant or nursing or if you have heart disease, high blood pressure, thyroid disease, or diabetes.

TARGET AILMENTS

Minor skin disorders

Cold sores

Uncomplicated hemorrhoidal itching and pain

SIDE EFFECTS

NOT SERIOUS
- Irritation of some mucous membranes; a burning sensation in the eyes

CALL YOUR DOCTOR IF THESE EFFECTS BECOME BOTHERSOME.

SERIOUS
- Allergic skin reactions, including large swellings, burning, or stinging
- Cardiovascular depression, indicated by low blood pressure, irregular heartbeat, paleness, or sweating (rare)
- Central nervous system toxicity (breathing difficulties, blurred vision, convulsions, dizziness, anxiety, ringing in the ears) caused by absorption of pramoxine through damaged skin (rare)

CALL YOUR DOCTOR RIGHT AWAY.

PROANTHOCYANIDIN

VITAL STATISTICS

OTHER NAMES
oligomeric procyanidolic complexes (OPC); procyanidolic oligomers (PCO)

GENERAL DESCRIPTION
Proanthocyanidin is among a group of naturally occurring plant compounds, called bioflavonoids, that have been found to protect and strengthen living tissue. A number of fruits—including blueberries, raspberries, cranberries, and cherries—contain proanthocyanidin. The substance is also found in pine bark, a fact that French explorer Jacques Cartier and his crew reportedly discovered in the 1500s while on expedition in Canada. With nothing to eat but biscuits and dried pork, the men began experiencing weakness, muscle aches, joint pains, and bruising. An Indian showed them how to make tea from pine bark. The explorers drank it, and their symptoms disappeared.

But by far the highest concentrations of proanthocyanidin are found in the seeds and skin of grapes. Recent research suggests that drinking red wine can help reduce the risk of cardiovascular disease, and many experts attribute these benefits to high levels of proanthocyanidin in the grapes.

Because it acts as an antioxidant, neutralizing "free radicals" that can harm the body, proanthocyanidin has been used in France for years as a treatment for blood vessel disorders. Considered an effective antihistamine and anti-inflammatory agent, the substance is also thought to protect and heal connective tissue, reduce inflammation, and stabilize collagen and elastin, thereby improving and preserving the elasticity of the skin.

PREPARATIONS
Proanthocyanidin is available in tablet and capsule form as a dietary supplement.

TARGET AILMENTS

Allergies that respond to antihistamines

Arthritis

Bruises

Gum disease

Phlebitis

Ulcers

Varicose veins and other vascular problems

SIDE EFFECTS
NONE EXPECTED

PSEUDOEPHEDRINE

VITAL STATISTICS

DRUG CLASS
Decongestants

BRAND NAMES
Actifed, Advil Cold and Sinus, Claritin-D, Comtrex Multi-Symptom Cold Reliever Tablets or Liquid, Contac, Drixoral, NyQuil, Pedia-Care (various forms), Sudafed, TheraFlu, Triaminic Nite Light, Triaminic Sore Throat Formula, Tylenol Allergy Sinus, Tylenol Cold (adults and children), Tylenol Sinus

OTHER DRUGS IN THIS CLASS
Rx: phenylpropanolamine
OTC: oxymetazoline, phenylephrine, phenyl-propanolamine

GENERAL DESCRIPTION
Pseudoephedrine is a synthetic decongestant drug modeled on the ephedrine found in plants of the *Ephedra* genus. The drug is used to treat congestion of the nasal, sinus, and Eustachian passages caused by colds, allergies, or related respiratory problems. It is often available in combination with analgesics, antihistamines, and expectorants. Pseudoephedrine is banned for use during athletic competitions. For more information, see Decongestants.

PRECAUTIONS

SPECIAL INFORMATION
- Some preparations that contain pseudoephedrine also contain antihistamines, which can cause other side effects, including drowsiness. See Antihistamines for further information.
- Check with your doctor before taking pseudoephedrine if you have cardiovascular disease (including angina, coronary artery disease, and hypertension), hyperthyroidism (overactive thyroid), prostate enlargement, diabetes, or glaucoma. The drug may exacerbate these conditions.

PSEUDOEPHEDRINE

POSSIBLE INTERACTIONS

Beta blockers: Pseudoephedrine can lessen the effectiveness of beta blockers, causing hypertension.

Digoxin: possible heart-rhythm problems.

High blood pressure drugs: decreased anti-hypertensive effect.

Levodopa (anti-Parkinsonism drug): increased risk of heart-rhythm problems.

Monoamine oxidase (MAO) inhibitors: increased stimulant action of pseudo-ephedrine, causing effects such as hyper-tension and heart-rhythm problems.

Rauwolfia: decreased effectiveness of pseudoephedrine.

Stimulants (such as other decongestants, am-phetamines, caffeine): increased stimulant effects, leading to excessive nervousness, in-somnia, irregular heart rhythm, or seizures.

Thyroid hormones: increased effects of both combined drugs. Your doctor may have to adjust the dosage of both medications.

Tricyclic antidepressants (such as amitripty-line): increased action of pseudoephedrine, making serious central nervous system side effects more likely.

TARGET AILMENTS

Nasal and sinus congestion

Congestion of Eustachian tubes, which join the ear with the nose and throat

SIDE EFFECTS

NOT SERIOUS

- Mild nervousness
- Mild restlessness
- Insomnia
- Dizziness
- Lightheadedness
- Nausea
- Dryness of mouth or nose
- Rebound congestion

CALL YOUR DOCTOR IF THESE EFFECTS CONTINUE OR BECOME BOTHERSOME.

SERIOUS

- Severe headache
- Nervousness
- Restlessness
- Pounding or irregular heartbeat
- High blood pressure
- Trouble breathing

CONTACT YOUR DOCTOR IMMEDIATELY.

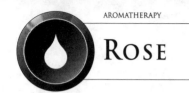

ROSE

LATIN NAME
Rosa damascena

VITAL STATISTICS

GENERAL DESCRIPTION

Rose oil, one of the most highly valued oils, is used both in aromatherapy and in making perfume. Much of the rose oil used in aromatherapy is produced from the damask rose, which originated in Syria and has been prized throughout the world for its sweet, soothing scent and the color and shape of its blooms, as well as for its therapeutic properties.

The petals and stamens are used to produce the oil, which is a pale yellow-green, oily in texture, and strongly scented. Rose water, also believed to have medicinal properties, is a by-product of this distillation process.

Rose oil is used externally to treat a wide variety of disorders, including respiratory infections, liver congestion, sensitive skin, broken capillaries, nausea, and stress. It is said to have antidepressant, antiseptic, astringent, and sedative properties and is considered a tonic for the heart, liver, stomach, and uterus.

PREPARATIONS

Rose water can be used as a gargle and rinse for sore throat and mouth ulcers. Cotton balls can be soaked in rose water and placed over the eyes to relieve fatigue and irritation.

BODY OIL: Combine 10 drops rose oil with 2 oz almond oil or aloe gel. Rub on the stomach, solar plexus, back of neck, temples, and other areas twice a day to relieve premenstrual or menopausal symptoms, to aid the liver, stomach, and circulatory system, or to help with skin problems.

Rose oil can be used in a diffuser to scent a room, sprinkled on a tissue and inhaled, or worn like perfume. For use in the bath, add 3 to 5 drops rose oil to the bathwater.

PRECAUTIONS

SPECIAL INFORMATION

Buy rose oil only from a reputable source. Because the oil is so expensive to produce, its purity may be compromised.

TARGET AILMENTS

Insomnia

Anxiety; depression

Nervous tension

Diminished sex drive

Loss of appetite

Nausea

Menstrual pain

Cough; hay fever

Sore throat

Mouth ulcers

Skin problems

Eye and eyelid complaints (rose water only)

SIDE EFFECTS

NONE EXPECTED

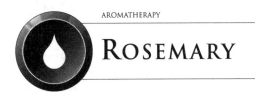

ROSEMARY

LATIN NAME
Rosmarinus officinalis

VITAL STATISTICS

GENERAL DESCRIPTION

This Mediterranean evergreen shrub has silvery green leaves and pale blue flowers. Its name in Latin means "dew of the sea." Rosemary had many symbolic associations in ancient times: love, death, and loyalty, for example. Today, it is one of the best known and most used of the aromatic herbs. Planted in the garden, rosemary discourages pests. The oil is colorless to pale yellow-green, and its scent is minty in oils of good quality.

A stimulant, rosemary is thought to invigorate the whole body and help eliminate toxins. Rosemary is said to have antiseptic and diuretic properties, and as an antispasmodic agent it is considered useful in relieving the pain of premenstrual tension and cramping, asthma, and rheumatic aches and pains.

PREPARATIONS

The best-quality oil is distilled from the flowering tops. It can also be distilled from the leaves and stems before the plant flowers, but the oil will be of an inferior quality.

FOR NEARLY ALL USES, rosemary can be applied to the skin: Add 15 drops of oil to 2 tbsp of vegetable or nut oil, or aloe gel. To add it to the bath, use 5 to 10 drops of oil. For treating hair loss and dandruff, add 20 drops of rosemary oil to 1 oz of shampoo, or add 7 to 10 drops of oil to 2 tbsp of aloe gel, then apply to scalp and leave on overnight.

TO INHALE, use a room diffuser or sprinkle a few drops of oil on a tissue or handkerchief and inhale the fragrance.

PRECAUTIONS

SPECIAL INFORMATION
- Avoid using rosemary during pregnancy.
- Do not use rosemary if you have epilepsy or high blood pressure.

TARGET AILMENTS

Indigestion and gas; constipation

Liver problems; fluid retention

Asthma and bronchitis; colds and flu

Depression

Rheumatism and arthritis

Mental fatigue; poor memory

Headache (apply diluted or undiluted to areas of pain)

Hair loss; dandruff

Low blood pressure

Varicose veins (skin application)

Irregular menstrual periods and menstrual pain

SIDE EFFECTS
NONE EXPECTED

ST.-JOHN'S-WORT

LATIN NAME
Hypericum perforatum

VITAL STATISTICS

GENERAL DESCRIPTION
Herbalists now know that the flowers of the plant called St.-John's-wort contain hypericin, a substance with germicidal, anti-inflammatory, and antidepressant properties. They also hold high concentrations of flavonoids, chemicals thought to boost the immune system. According to ancient healing wisdom, because the plant (*wort* means "plant" in Old English) seemed to resemble skin, and because, when pinched, it produces a red oil, it was considered an ideal remedy for all manner of flesh wounds. Today, it is generally used for the soothing effect it is said to have on injured nerves.

PREPARATIONS
Over the counter:
Available as dried leaves and flowers, tinctures, extract, oil, ointment, capsules, and prepared tea.

At home:
TEA: Add 1 to 2 tsp dried herb to 1 cup boiling water; steep covered for 15 minutes. Drink up to 3 cups a day.
OIL: Use a commercial preparation, or make by soaking the flowers in almond or olive oil until the oil turns bright red.
OINTMENT: Use a commercial preparation, or make by warming the leaves in hot petroleum jelly or a mixture of beeswax and almond oil.
FRESH: Apply crushed leaves and flowers to cleaned wounds.
TINCTURE: Add ¼ to 1 tsp to an 8-oz glass of water and drink daily.
Consult a qualified practitioner for the dosage appropriate for your specific condition.

PRECAUTIONS

SPECIAL INFORMATION
- Consult a doctor or herbalist before using St.-John's-wort.
- Use of this herb by children for more than seven to 10 days should be done in conjunction with a healthcare practitioner.

POSSIBLE INTERACTIONS
Amino acids tryptophan and tyrosine; amphetamines; asthma inhalants; beer, coffee, wine; chocolate, fava beans, salami, smoked or pickled foods, and yogurt; cold or hay fever medicines; diet pills; narcotics; nasal decongestants: possible high blood pressure and nausea.

TARGET AILMENTS

Use externally for:

Wounds, including cuts, abrasions, burns; scar tissue

Take internally, in consultation with a herbalist or a doctor, for:

Depression

SIDE EFFECTS

SERIOUS
- High blood pressure; headaches; stiff neck
- Nausea; vomiting
- Worsening of sunburn in the fair-skinned; blistering after sun exposure.

CALL YOUR DOCTOR IMMEDIATELY.

SAW PALMETTO

LATIN NAME
Serenoa repens

VITAL STATISTICS

GENERAL DESCRIPTION

An extract made from the berries of this shrub is used to strengthen and treat problems with the male reproductive system. It is particularly recommended for benign enlargement of the prostate gland, which is indicated by urination difficulties and can lead to bladder infections and kidney problems. Common among men over 50, the condition is thought to be caused by an accumulation of a testosterone derivative called dihydrotestosterone; saw palmetto appears to block the production of this chemical.

Saw palmetto has also been used as an expectorant, diuretic, tonic, antiseptic, sedative, and digestive aid. It is native to the sandy coast of the southeastern United States, where the plant reaches a height of about 10 feet.

PREPARATIONS

Over the counter:
Available as fresh or dried berries and in powder or capsule form. Gel capsules are preferable to tea or tincture, because the active ingredients of the herb are fat soluble and do not dissolve well in water.

At home:
INFUSION: If you have fresh berries, prepare by steeping covered ½ to 1 tsp berries per cup of boiling water for 10 minutes. Drink 6 oz, two or three times a day.
DECOCTION: Add ½ to 1 tsp dried berries to 1 cup water, bring to a boil, and simmer covered for 5 minutes. Drink three times daily.
TINCTURE: Drink ¼ to ½ tsp in water two or three times daily.
Consult a practitioner for the dosage appropriate for you and your condition.

PRECAUTIONS

☠ WARNING

Do not substitute saw palmetto for medical treatment. Although this herb is thought to be effective for treating an enlarged prostate, it has no known effect against prostate cancer. Because the symptoms of prostate enlargement and prostate cancer are similar, men should see a doctor when they have urological symptoms such as urine retention, dribbling, and passage of blood in the urine.

SPECIAL INFORMATION

This herb should not be used with children unless it is prescribed by a healthcare practitioner who is knowledgeable about herbs.

POSSIBLE INTERACTIONS

Combining saw palmetto with other herbs may necessitate a lower dosage.

TARGET AILMENTS

Use internally for treatment of:

Benign prostatic hyperplasia (enlargement of the prostate gland)

Nasal congestion

Bronchitis

Coughs due to colds

SIDE EFFECTS
NONE EXPECTED

SELENIUM

VITAL STATISTICS

GENERAL DESCRIPTION

An antioxidant, selenium protects cells and tissues from damage wrought by free radicals. Because its antioxidant effects complement those of vitamin E, the two are said to potentiate, or reinforce, each other. Selenium also supports immune function and neutralizes certain poisonous substances, such as cadmium, mercury, and arsenic, that may be ingested or inhaled. Although its full therapeutic value is unknown, adequate selenium levels may help combat arthritis, deter heart disease, and prevent cancer.

Very little selenium is required to maintain good health, and most people get adequate amounts through diet alone. Some multinutrients contain selenium, but always in small, safe amounts.

RDA

Men: 70 mcg
Women: 55 mcg
Pregnant women: 65 mcg

NATURAL SOURCES

Whole grains, asparagus, garlic, eggs, and mushrooms are typically good sources, as are lean meats and seafood.

PRECAUTIONS

☠ WARNING

Selenium can be toxic in extremely high doses, causing hair loss, nail problems, accelerated tooth decay, and swelling of the fingers, among other symptoms.

SPECIAL INFORMATION

High-dose supplements such as selenium citrate and selenium picolinate should be taken only if prescribed by a doctor.

TARGET AILMENTS

Arthritis

Cancer

Heart disease

Immune problems

SIDE EFFECTS
NONE EXPECTED

SHARK CARTILAGE

VITAL STATISTICS

GENERAL DESCRIPTION

Shark cartilage is a nutritional supplement that has generated considerable controversy. Proponents say the substance has numerous potential uses, from stimulating the immune system to treating cancer. Some claim it is an effective anti-inflammatory that can relieve joint swelling, pain, and stiffness. Critics, on the other hand, say there is no scientific evidence of its effectiveness. Even manufacturers of the supplement acknowledge that, although studies are encouraging, the usefulness of shark cartilage as a cancer treatment has not been scientifically proved.

Shark cartilage is thought to have medicinal value largely because of two characteristics of the creatures themselves: Sharks have no bones, only cartilage, and they rarely get cancer. One theory is that something in the cartilage blocks the formation of new blood vessels, which tumors need in order to grow.

PREPARATIONS

Shark cartilage is sold in the United States in tablet form as a dietary supplement.

PRECAUTIONS

☠ WARNING

This supplement should never be substituted for conventional cancer treatment. Because little is known about the potential effects of shark cartilage, do not take this supplement if you are pregnant.

SPECIAL INFORMATION

Taken at therapeutic levels, shark cartilage provides extremely high doses of calcium. Have your blood calcium level monitored if you are taking large amounts of this supplement.

TARGET AILMENTS
Joint pain
Stiffness
Swelling

SIDE EFFECTS
NONE EXPECTED

SIMETHICONE

VITAL STATISTICS

DRUG CLASS
Antigas Drugs

BRAND NAMES
Tums Antigas/Antacid formula; some types of Mylanta; Mylanta Gas; some types of Maalox

GENERAL DESCRIPTION
Simethicone is an antigas drug used to relieve the pain, cramping, bloating, intestinal pressure, and "full" sensation that accompany flatulence, or gas. Gas can build up in the gastrointestinal tract as a result of excessive swallowing of air or from eating foods the body does not tolerate well.

The defoaming properties of simethicone act in the gastrointestinal tract to disperse gas bubbles and to prevent their formation. The drug changes the surface tension of small gas bubbles in the stomach, causing them to coalesce and form larger ones. These larger bubbles are more easily expelled through belching or passing flatus. Simethicone is often combined with antacids for the dual relief of gas and heartburn.

Simethicone tablets should be chewed thoroughly before swallowing.

PRECAUTIONS

☠ WARNING
Do not take this drug if you have kidney disease.

SPECIAL INFORMATION
- Simethicone is nontoxic; when used as indicated, the drug produces no side effects. A possible adverse effect could include excessive expulsion of gas in belching or flatus.
- The adult dosages of this drug are not recommended for treating infant colic. Infant drops are available, but check with your pediatrician for guidance on their use.
- Do not take this medication for more than two weeks.
- Do not exceed the recommended dosage.

POSSIBLE INTERACTIONS
Although unlikely, this drug may interact with some medications. Check with your doctor before using a product containing simethicone if you are taking other drugs.

TARGET AILMENTS
Symptoms of gas (bloating, abdominal cramps, intestinal pressure, fullness)

Postoperative gaseous distention

SIDE EFFECTS
NONE EXPECTED

SMOKING CESSATION DRUGS

VITAL STATISTICS

GENERIC NAME
nicotine

BRAND NAMES
Rx: Nicotrol NS (nasal spray)
OTC: NicoDerm CQ (transdermal), Nicorette (chewing gum); Nicotrol (transdermal)

GENERAL DESCRIPTION
Smoking cessation drugs, available in the form of flavored chewing gum, transdermal (skin) patches, and nasal spray, are used to reduce nicotine craving and withdrawal effects in people who want to stop smoking. These aids serve as temporary alternative sources of nicotine and are most useful to those smokers who have a strong physical dependence on the drug.

Nicotine acts on the peripheral and central nervous systems, producing stimulant and depressant effects. By slowly reducing nicotine intake, these products can lessen the physical effects of smoking withdrawal, such as irritability, nervousness, drowsiness, fatigue, headache, and nicotine craving. There is no evidence that nicotine replacement drugs work unless the smoker also participates in a medically supervised stop-smoking program.

PRECAUTIONS

☠ WARNING
Extremely high doses of nicotine can produce toxic symptoms; nicotine overdose can be fatal. Because of the risk of overdose, do not smoke when using a medicinal form of nicotine.

SPECIAL INFORMATION
- In order for smoking cessation drugs to be safe and effective, stop smoking completely at the beginning of treatment. This is also essential because of the risk of nicotine overdose.
- Call your doctor immediately if you have any of the following symptoms of toxic nicotine overdose: nausea, vomiting, abdominal cramps, diarrhea, dizziness, sweating, hearing or vision problems, confusion, weakness.
- Nicotine replacement products should not be used by nonsmokers or others who are not addicted to the drug.
- Do not use smoking cessation drugs if you have had an allergic reaction to them before. Consult your doctor if you have angina or an abnormal heart rhythm; have had a recent heart attack; or are pregnant, planning a pregnancy, or nursing.

125

CONTINUED

SMOKING CESSATION DRUGS

- Tell your doctor if you have diabetes, high blood pressure, skin disease, overactive thyroid, adrenaline-producing tumors, peptic ulcer, or liver or kidney disease, or if you get rashes from adhesive bandages or tape.
- Tell your doctor what other medications you are taking. Changes in nicotine levels may require dosage adjustments for other drugs, especially those affecting the nervous system.
- Nicotine can be very harmful to children and pets. Be sure to dispose of used patches carefully, and keep nasal sprays out of reach at all times.
- Do not use smoking cessation drugs for more than 12 to 20 weeks (depending on the system) if you have succeeded in stopping smoking. Continued use can be harmful and addictive.

POSSIBLE INTERACTIONS

Bronchodilators, insulin, propoxyphene, and propranolol and other beta-adrenergic blockers: you may need decreased amounts of these drugs when you stop smoking.

Isoproterenol, phenylephrine: you may need increased amounts of these drugs when you stop smoking.

TARGET AILMENTS

Smoking cessation

Nicotine withdrawal

SIDE EFFECTS

NOT SERIOUS

- Mild, temporary irritation (redness, tingling, itchiness) at a patch site
- Fast heartbeat
- Coughing; dry mouth
- Muscle or joint pain
- Hot feeling at the back of the throat or nose; sneezing; watery eyes; runny nose (nasal spray)

CALL YOUR DOCTOR IF THESE SYMPTOMS PERSIST OR ARE BOTHERSOME.

- Increased appetite
- Mild headache, irritability, or nervousness
- Unusual dreams

THESE ARE SYMPTOMS OF NICOTINE WITHDRAWAL.

SERIOUS

- Chest pain
- Irregular heartbeat
- Dizziness
- Allergic reactions (hives, rash, swelling)
- Tingling in the arms or legs
- Tingling, burning, numbness in the nose, throat, or mouth (nasal spray)

CHECK WITH YOUR DOCTOR. ALSO SEE SIGNS OF OVERDOSE UNDER SPECIAL INFORMATION.

SOYBEAN MILK

GENERAL DESCRIPTION

As more people in the United States cut down on the amount of red meat in their diet, soy is rapidly gaining popularity. The main reason is that soy products, including soybean milk, are among the few plant foods that provide complete proteins, which are essential for a healthy diet and can be more difficult to obtain in a diet that includes little meat.

Not only is soy a good source of protein, it also contains chemical compounds that can play a role in fighting cancer. These compounds are plant-based hormones called phytoestrogens. High levels of a specific class of phytoestrogens known as isoflavones are found in soy products. Isoflavones play two roles in preventing cancer. They act as antioxidants, protecting body cells from the harmful effects of "free radicals," or unstable oxygen by-products that can damage cell DNA. Isoflavones also act as antimutagens, preventing cell mutations that can develop into cancerous tumors.

Some research also suggests isoflavones may prevent the negative effects of naturally occurring estrogen hormones that play a role in the development of breast, ovarian, and endometrial cancers. The rates of breast and prostate cancers are far lower in Asian countries, where soy-based diets are the norm. The phytoestrogens in soy may also help lessen the severity of symptoms for women going through menopause. Many experts suggest that women approaching menopause include soy in their daily diets.

In addition to these benefits, soy can help reduce blood cholesterol levels. Soy is also a good source of folate, iron, and magnesium as well as calcium, which can help prevent osteoporosis.

Soybean milk, or soya milk, is a particularly good choice for people who are lactose intolerant, since it contains no lactose, a difficult-to-digest milk sugar that some people must avoid. There's no cholesterol in soya milk, although it does contain fat. Regular formulas of soya milk have nearly as much fat as 2 percent milk; light versions contain about as much as 1 percent milk. The taste can be a little chalky.

PREPARATIONS

Soya milk is available in the United States at health food stores and in a number of grocery stores. The taste varies from brand to brand.

TARGET AILMENTS

High cholesterol

Lactose intolerance

Osteoporosis

Breast, ovarian, and endometrial cancers (risk reduction)

SIDE EFFECTS
NONE EXPECTED

TOLNAFTATE

VITAL STATISTICS

DRUG CLASS
Antifungal Drugs

BRAND NAME
Tinactin

OTHER DRUGS IN THIS CLASS
Rx: clotrimazole, fluconazole, ketoconazole, miconazole, terconazole
OTC: clotrimazole, miconazole, undecylenate

GENERAL DESCRIPTION
Tolnaftate, available in topical aerosol, powder, cream, gel, or solution form, is used to treat several types of superficial fungal infections. It can also help prevent the development of some types of athlete's foot. Tolnaftate is not an effective treatment for bacterial or yeast infections (candidiasis). For more information, see Antifungal Drugs.

PRECAUTIONS

SPECIAL INFORMATION
- Do not use on children under age two or for diaper rash without consulting your doctor.
- Contact your doctor if your symptoms worsen or do not improve within 10 days.
- Do not allow the medication to come in contact with your eyes.
- Because it lacks antibacterial properties, tolnaftate is most effective for the dry, scaly type of athlete's foot.
- Although it may sting slightly when first applied, tolnaftate can be applied to broken skin.

- To prevent reinfection of fungal infections involving the feet or genitals, wear cotton rather than synthetic-fiber socks or underwear during treatment.
- Avoid wearing tight underwear if you have jock itch.

POSSIBLE INTERACTIONS
None expected.

TARGET AILMENTS

Jock itch

Body ringworm

White-brown skin patches (a ringworm infection known as tinea versicolor)

Athlete's foot

SIDE EFFECTS

NOT SERIOUS
- Skin may become slightly irritated at the site of application

IF THIS BECOMES BOTHERSOME, DISCONTINUE USE AND CONSULT YOUR DOCTOR.

TOPICAL ANTIBIOTICS

VITAL STATISTICS

GENERIC NAMES

Rx: chlorhexidine (for gums); mupirocin (for skin); combination of neomycin, polymyxin B, and hydrocortisone (antibiotic-corticosteroid for ears)
OTC: bacitracin, neomycin, polymyxin B

GENERAL DESCRIPTION

Topical antibiotics are used to prevent or clear up bacterial infections of the skin, ears, or gums. They should never be used interchangeably; drugs for the skin, for example, should not be applied to the ears or mouth. Each drug is effective against a specific group of bacteria. For self-treatment of minor skin wounds, it may therefore be useful to choose an over-the-counter product that combines two or more antibacterial ingredients.

Over-the-counter topical antibiotics are available in an ointment base that helps close and soothe wounds. In general, though, OTC drugs are used to guard against possible infections. Once a skin infection is under way, your doctor may prescribe a stronger medication.

PRECAUTIONS

SPECIAL INFORMATION

- Check with your doctor if you notice no improvement after using these medications for two or three days.
- Prolonged use of a prescription topical antibiotic may result in fungal superinfection.
- The use of topical antibiotics increases the risk of kidney damage or hearing loss in people with impaired kidney function who are already taking nephrotoxic medicines.
- If you are pregnant or nursing, check with your doctor before using.

POSSIBLE INTERACTIONS

Aminoglycosides: possible hypersensitivity reaction and toxicity, leading to permanent deafness if combined with neomycin, which is also an aminoglycoside.

TARGET AILMENTS

Minor cuts, scrapes, and burns (bacitracin, neomycin, polymyxin B, to prevent bacterial infection)

Gingivitis (chlorhexidine)

Impetigo (mupirocin)

External ear canal infections (neomycin, polymyxin B, and hydrocortisone in combination)

SIDE EFFECTS

CHECK INDIVIDUAL PRODUCT LABELS FOR POSSIBLE SIDE EFFECTS.

VAGINAL ANTIFUNGAL DRUGS

DRUG CLASS
Antifungal Drugs

GENERIC NAMES
Rx: clotrimazole, fluconazole, miconazole, terconazole
OTC: clotrimazole, miconazole

GENERAL DESCRIPTION
Vaginal antifungal drugs are commonly prescribed for vaginal yeast infections. They work by damaging the membranes of fungal cells and inhibiting the enzyme activity essential for the cells' growth and reproduction. The drugs are available in the form of vaginal creams and suppositories. For more information, see Antifungal Drugs.

PRECAUTIONS

SPECIAL INFORMATION
- If you are pregnant or nursing, do not use a vaginal antifungal medication without consulting your doctor.
- Do not use if you have a fever above 100°F; abdominal, shoulder, or back pain; or a malodorous vaginal discharge.
- Be sure to use these medications for the prescribed amount of time, even during menstruation or if your symptoms abate.
- If you are using a vaginal cream, protect clothing from possible soiling by wearing panty liners or sanitary napkins.
- Avoid possible reinfection by wearing cotton rather than synthetic-fiber underwear.
- Refrain from sexual activity during treatment to avoid possible transmission and reinfection. Also, be aware that some vaginal antifungal preparations contain a vegetable oil base that might weaken latex condoms, diaphragms, or cervical caps.
- If your male partner has any penile discomfort, burning, irritation, or itchiness, he may require simultaneous treatment for infection. He should consult his doctor.
- Douching may or may not be advised while using this medication; consult your doctor.
- If your symptoms do not show improvement within three to seven days, consult your doctor.
- If your symptoms return within two months, see your doctor; you may be pregnant or have a serious disorder, such as diabetes or an HIV infection.

TARGET AILMENTS

Yeast infections (candidiasis) of the vulva and vagina

SIDE EFFECTS

NOT SERIOUS
- Headaches; mild abdominal or stomach cramps; irritation to the sexual partner's penis (rare)

CALL YOUR DOCTOR IF THESE SYMPTOMS CONTINUE OR ARE TROUBLESOME.

SERIOUS
- Vaginal burning, itching, or discharge; skin rash, hives, or other skin irritation

DISCONTINUE THE MEDICATION AND CONTACT YOUR DOCTOR.

VALERIAN

LATIN NAME
Valeriana officinalis

VITAL STATISTICS

GENERAL DESCRIPTION

Valerian root has been used for more than 1,000 years for its calming qualities, and recent research has confirmed its efficacy and safety as a mild tranquilizer and sleep aid. For sufferers of insomnia, valerian has been found to hasten the onset of sleep, improve sleep quality, and reduce nighttime awakenings. Unlike barbiturates or benzodiazepines, prescribed amounts leave no morning grogginess and do not interfere with the vivid dreaming sleep known as REM sleep. It is not habit forming and produces no withdrawal symptoms when discontinued. The plant is a hardy perennial that reaches a height of about five feet. As the roots dry, they develop an unpleasant odor compared by one herbalist to that of dirty socks. Most people add sugar or honey to make valerian tea more palatable.

PREPARATIONS

Over the counter:
Valerian is widely available dried or as capsules, tinctures, and teas.

At home:
TEA: Steep covered 2 tsp dried, chopped root in 1 cup boiling water. Let stand covered 8 to 12 hours. Or simmer covered 2 tsp root in 8 oz water for 10 minutes. Drink 1 cup before bed.
Consult a qualified practitioner for the dosage appropriate for you and the specific condition being treated.

PRECAUTIONS

SPECIAL INFORMATION

- Do not take valerian with conventional tranquilizers or sedatives, because of possible additive effects.
- Paradoxically, valerian may produce excitability in some people.
- Because valerian is a sedative, avoid driving until you know how the herb affects you.

POSSIBLE INTERACTIONS

Combining valerian with other herbs may necessitate a lower dosage.

TARGET AILMENTS

Insomnia; anxiety, nervousness, anxiety-induced heart palpitations; headache; intestinal pains; menstrual cramps

SIDE EFFECTS

NOT SERIOUS

- Mild headache; upset stomach

REDUCE DOSAGE; LET YOUR DOCTOR KNOW IF PROBLEMS PERSIST.

SERIOUS

- More severe headache; restlessness; nausea; morning grogginess; blurred vision (using too much valerian)

CONTACT YOUR DOCTOR, WHO WILL PROBABLY TELL YOU TO TAKE LESS OR STOP USING THE HERB.

VITAMIN A

VITAL STATISTICS

OTHER NAMES
retinene, retinoic acid, retinol, retinyl palmitate

GENERAL DESCRIPTION
The first vitamin ever discovered, vitamin A is essential for good vision—especially in dim light—and for healthy skin, hair, and mucous membranes of the nose, throat, respiratory system, and digestive system. This vitamin is also necessary for the proper growth and development of bones and teeth. It stimulates the healing of wounds and is used to treat some skin disorders. Beta carotene, the precursor to vitamin A, is a carotenoid, a type of pigment found in plants. Your skin stores beta carotene, and your body metabolizes it to produce vitamin A as needed. Excess beta carotene, along with other carotenoids such as alpha carotene, acts as an antioxidant and supports immune function, so it increases your resistance to infection; it may help prevent some cancers and vision problems such as night blindness. Beta carotene may also help lower cholesterol levels and reduce the risk of heart disease.

RDA
Men: 5,000 IU (or 3 mg beta carotene)
Women: 4,000 IU (or 2.4 mg beta carotene)

NATURAL SOURCES
Vitamin A is present in orange and yellow vegetables and fruits such as dried apricots, sweet potatoes, and yams; dark green leafy vegetables such as broccoli, collard and mustard greens, and kale; chili peppers; whole milk, cream, and butter; and organ meats such as liver.

PRECAUTIONS

☠ WARNING
Because it is fat soluble, vitamin A is stored in the body long term, and toxicity is possible if one uses high doses over a long period of time. Beta carotene does not have associated toxicity, even in high doses.

Pregnant women or women who may become pregnant should avoid supplementation. Doses over 10,000 IU during pregnancy may result in birth defects.

SPECIAL INFORMATION
Too much vitamin A can cause headaches; insomnia; restlessness; vision problems; nausea; dry, flaking skin; or an enlarged liver or spleen.

TARGET AILMENTS

Cancer

Heart disease

High cholesterol

Immune problems

Vision problems

Wounds

Viral illnesses

Vaginal candidiasis

SIDE EFFECTS
NONE EXPECTED
AT RECOMMENDED LEVELS.

VITAMIN B₁ (THIAMINE)

VITAL STATISTICS

OTHER NAME
thiamine

GENERAL DESCRIPTION
Thiamine is sometimes called the energy vitamin because it is needed to metabolize carbohydrates, fats, and proteins and helps convert excess glucose into stored fat. Vitamin B_1 also ensures proper nerve-impulse transmission and contributes to maintaining normal appetite, muscle tone, and mental health. In the 1930s thiamine was discovered to be the cure for the crippling and potentially fatal disease beriberi. Now that rice, flour, and bread are generally enriched with thiamine, beriberi is relatively rare.

RDA
Men: 1.5 mg
Women: 1.1 mg

NATURAL SOURCES
A diet that regularly includes lean pork, milk, whole grains, peas, beans, peanuts, or soybeans generally provides enough thiamine.

PRECAUTIONS

☠ WARNING
Alcohol suppresses thiamine absorption; for this reason and because they typically have poor diets, alcoholics are likely to be deficient in thiamine and other nutrients.

SPECIAL INFORMATION
- Athletes, laborers, pregnant women, and other people who burn great amounts of energy may require more than the adult RDA of thiamine.
- Mild deficiency may cause fatigue, loss of appetite, nausea, moodiness, confusion, anemia, and possibly heart arrhythmias. To increase thiamine levels, try changing your diet or taking a multivitamin instead of thiamine supplements.
- Large doses up to 100 mg of thiamine may alleviate itching from insect bites; otherwise, megasupplements are not known to be either harmful or helpful.
- Very large doses may cause nervousness, itching, flushing, or tachycardia in sensitive people.

TARGET AILMENTS

Anemia

Fatigue

SIDE EFFECTS
NONE EXPECTED

VITAMIN B₂

VITAL STATISTICS

OTHER NAME
riboflavin

GENERAL DESCRIPTION
Like other members of the vitamin B complex, riboflavin helps produce energy from carbohydrates, fats, and proteins. Riboflavin also promotes healthy skin, hair, nails, and mucous membranes; aids the production of red blood cells, corticosteroids, and thyroid hormones; and is required for the proper function of the nerves, eyes, and adrenal glands. It is often used to treat acne, anemia, cataracts, and depression.

RDA
Men: 1.7 mg
Women: 1.3 mg
Pregnant women: 1.6 mg

NATURAL SOURCES
Lean organ meats, enriched bread and flour, cheese, yogurt, eggs, almonds, soybean products such as tofu, and green leafy vegetables—especially broccoli—are good sources. Store these foods in the dark, because vitamin B₂ breaks down in sunlight.

PRECAUTIONS

☠ WARNING
Alcoholics and elderly people are susceptible to riboflavin deficiency: The signs include oily, dry, scaly skin rash; sores, especially on the lips and corners of the mouth; a swollen, red, painful tongue; sensitivity to light; and burning or red, itchy eyes.

SPECIAL INFORMATION
- Although vitamin B₂ supplements are available, they provide far more riboflavin than anyone needs. Diet changes are better, or take a multivitamin supplement. It is best to take the supplements with food, which increases their absorption tremendously compared with taking the tablets alone.
- A well-balanced diet provides most people with adequate riboflavin, although athletes and others who need a great deal of energy may require more than the RDA.

TARGET AILMENTS

Fatigue

Depression

Skin problems

Vision problems

SIDE EFFECTS
NONE EXPECTED

VITAMIN B₆

VITAL STATISTICS

OTHER NAME
pyridoxine

GENERAL DESCRIPTION
Vitamin B₆ encompasses a family of compounds that includes pyridoxine, pyridoxamine, and pyridoxal. This vitamin supports immune function, nerve-impulse transmission (especially in the brain), energy metabolism, and red blood cell synthesis. Prescribed as a drug, vitamin B₆ can sometimes alleviate carpal tunnel syndrome, infant seizures, and premenstrual syndrome.

RDA
Men: 2 mg
Women: 1.6 mg
Pregnant women: 2.2 mg

NATURAL SOURCES
Brown rice, lean meats, poultry, fish, bananas, avocados, whole grains, corn, and nuts are rich in vitamin B₆.

PRECAUTIONS

☠ WARNING
Taking too much or too little vitamin B₆ can impair nerve function and mental health. If high levels (2,000 mg to 5,000 mg) are taken for several months, vitamin B₆ can become habit forming and may induce sleepiness as well as tingling, numb hands and feet. These symptoms will most likely disappear when the vitamin B₆ intake is reduced, and there is usually no permanent damage.

SPECIAL INFORMATION

- People most likely to be at risk for vitamin B₆ deficiency include anyone with a malabsorption problem such as lactose intolerance or celiac disease; diabetic or elderly people; and women who are pregnant, nursing, or taking oral contraceptives.
- Severe deficiency is rare. Mild deficiency may cause acne and inflamed skin, insomnia, muscle weakness, peripheral neuropathy or paresthesias that can mimic carpal tunnel syndrome, nausea, irritability, depression, and fatigue. For mild deficiency, a daily multivitamin supplement is usually recommended to boost low vitamin B₆ levels.

TARGET AILMENTS

Carpal tunnel syndrome

Depression

Fatigue

Immune problems

Premenstrual syndrome

Skin problems

SIDE EFFECTS
NONE EXPECTED

VITAMIN B₁₂

VITAL STATISTICS

OTHER NAME
cobalamin

GENERAL DESCRIPTION
Vitamin B_{12} is the largest and most complex family of the B vitamins; it includes several chemical compounds known as cobalamins. Cyanocobalamin, the stablest form, is the one most likely to be found in supplements. Like other B vitamins, B_{12} is important for converting fats, carbohydrates, and protein into energy, and assisting in the synthesis of red blood cells. It is critical for producing the genetic materials RNA and DNA as well as myelin, a fatty substance that forms a protective sheath around nerves.

Unlike other B vitamins, vitamin B_{12} needs several hours to be absorbed. Excess vitamin B_{12} is excreted in urine, even though a backup supply can be stored for several years in the liver. Vitamin B_{12} is considered nontoxic, even when taken at several times the RDA.

RDA
Adults: 2 mcg
Pregnant women: 2.2 mcg

NATURAL SOURCES
Vitamin B_{12} is not produced by plants but is supplied through animal products such as organ meats, fish, eggs, and dairy products.

TARGET AILMENTS

Anemia

Depression

Fatigue

PRECAUTIONS

SPECIAL INFORMATION
- High doses of folic acid (vitamin B_9) can decrease levels of B_{12}.
- Dietary deficiency is uncommon and is usually limited to alcoholics, strict vegetarians, and pregnant or nursing women—who should take supplements. More often, deficiency stems from an inability to absorb the vitamin, a problem that may occur for years before symptoms show; it tends to affect the elderly, those who have had stomach surgery, or people who have a disease of malabsorption, such as colitis.
- Signs of vitamin B_{12} deficiency include a sore tongue, weakness, weight loss, body odor, back pains, and tingling arms and legs. Severe deficiency leads to pernicious anemia, causing fatigue, a tendency to bleed, lemon yellow pallor, abdominal pain, stiff arms and legs, irritability, and depression.
- Without treatment, pernicious anemia can lead to permanent nerve damage and possibly death; the disease can be controlled, although not cured, with regular injections of B_{12}.
- Lack of calcium, vitamin B_6, or iron may also interfere with the normal absorption of vitamin B_{12}.

SIDE EFFECTS
NONE EXPECTED

VITAMIN C

VITAL STATISTICS

OTHER NAME
ascorbic acid

GENERAL DESCRIPTION
Vitamin C is well known for its ability to prevent and treat scurvy, a disease that causes swollen and bleeding gums, aching bones and muscles, and in some cases even death. Connective tissue throughout the body is made of collagen, which depends on vitamin C for its production. In this role, vitamin C helps heal wounds, burns, bruises, and broken bones. As a powerful antioxidant and immune system booster, vitamin C may alleviate the pain of rheumatoid arthritis, protect against atherosclerosis and heart disease, and help prevent some forms of cancer, and has the reputed potential (yet unproved) to prevent the common cold. More than the RDA may be needed under conditions of physical or emotional stress.

Because it is water soluble, excess vitamin C is excreted in the urine, so large amounts of it may usually be taken without fear of toxicity. Doses larger than 1,000 mg a day have been suggested for preventing cancer, infections including the common cold, and other ailments.

RDA
Adults: 60 mg
Pregnant women: 70 mg

NATURAL SOURCES
Sources of vitamin C include citrus fruits, rose hips, bell peppers, strawberries, broccoli, cantaloupes, tomatoes, and leafy greens.

PRECAUTIONS

☠ WARNING
In some people, large doses of vitamin C may induce such side effects as nausea, diarrhea, reduced selenium and copper absorption, excessive iron absorption, increased kidney stone formation, and a false-positive reaction to diabetes tests.

SPECIAL INFORMATION
- Vitamin C breaks down faster than any other vitamin, so it is best to eat fruits and vegetables when fresh and to cook them minimally or not at all.
- Slight vitamin C deficiency is fairly common, although severe deficiencies are rare in the United States today. Symptoms of deficiency include weight loss, fatigue, bleeding gums, easy bruising, reduced resistance to colds and other infections, and wounds and fractures that are slow to heal.

TARGET AILMENTS
Cancer

Heart disease

Immune problems

Wounds

SIDE EFFECTS
NONE EXPECTED

VITAMIN D

VITAL STATISTICS

OTHER NAMES
cholecalciferol, ergocalciferol

GENERAL DESCRIPTION
Vitamin D not only promotes healthy bones and teeth by regulating the absorption and balance of calcium and phosphorus but also fosters normal muscle contraction and nerve function. Vitamin D prevents rickets, a disease of calcium-deprived bone that results in bowlegs, knock-knees, and other bone defects. Vitamin D supplements may help treat psoriasis and slow or even reverse some cancers, such as myeloid leukemia.

RDA
Adults: 200 IU (5 mcg)
Children, adolescents, and pregnant women: 400 IU (10 mcg)

NATURAL SOURCES
Fatty fish such as herring, salmon, and tuna, followed by dairy products, are the richest natural sources of this nutrient. Few other foods naturally contain vitamin D, but 10 minutes in the midday summer sun enables the body to produce about 200 IU of it. Milk, breakfast cereals, and infant formulas are fortified with vitamin D.

PRECAUTIONS

☠ WARNING
Vitamin D is fat soluble; excess amounts of it are stored in the body. Because of its potentially toxic effects, vitamin D should not be taken in supplements of more than 400 IU daily unless prescribed by a doctor.

SPECIAL INFORMATION
- In adults, vitamin D deficiency can cause nervousness and diarrhea, insomnia, muscle twitches, and bone weakening, and it may worsen osteoporosis.
- Too much vitamin D raises the calcium level in the blood, which in turn may induce headaches, nausea, loss of appetite, excessive thirst, muscle weakness, and even heart, liver, or kidney damage as calcium deposits accumulate in soft tissue.
- In some latitudes, people don't get enough sunshine and cannot make enough vitamin D for several months of the year; those people should ensure that they get enough through diet or through supplements in the amount of 400 IU to 800 IU per day. Supplements over 400 IU per day should be prescribed by a doctor, however.

TARGET AILMENTS
Cancer

Skin problems

SIDE EFFECTS
NONE EXPECTED

VITAMIN E

VITAL STATISTICS

OTHER NAME
alpha-tocopherol

GENERAL DESCRIPTION
Vitamin E encompasses a family of compounds called tocopherols, of which alpha-tocopherol is the most common. It is required for proper function of the immune system, endocrine system, and sex glands. As a powerful antioxidant, it prevents unstable molecules known as free radicals from damaging cells and tissues. In this capacity, vitamin E deters atherosclerosis, accelerates the healing of wounds, protects lung tissue from inhaled pollutants, may reduce risk for heart disease, and may prevent premature skin aging. Researchers suspect that vitamin E has other beneficial effects ranging from preventing cancer and cataracts to alleviating rheumatoid arthritis and a skin disorder associated with lupus.

Because of its many suggested therapeutic roles, vitamin E is popular as an oral supplement and an ingredient of skin-care products. Although it is fat soluble, vitamin E is considered nontoxic because it does no harm except in extremely high doses.

RDA
Women: 12 IU (8 mg)
Men and pregnant or nursing women: 15 IU (10 mg)

NATURAL SOURCES
Vegetable oils, nuts, dark green leafy vegetables, organ meats, seafood, eggs, and avocados are rich food sources of vitamin E.

PRECAUTIONS

SPECIAL INFORMATION
Symptoms of vitamin E deficiency, such as fluid retention and hemolytic anemia, are rare in adults but are sometimes seen in premature infants.

TARGET AILMENTS
Arthritis

Heart disease

Skin problems

Wounds

SIDE EFFECTS
NONE EXPECTED

WHEAT GERM

VITAL STATISTICS

GENERAL DESCRIPTION

Wheat germ, the heart of the wheat berry, is the most healthful part of the grain. It contains vitamins B and E, protein, iron, calcium, copper, magnesium, zinc, and potassium.

Wheat germ is a good source of fiber, which can relieve constipation and may reduce the risk of developing colon and rectal cancer. A quarter cup contains 40 percent of the recommended daily allowance of vitamin E. In addition, including wheat germ as part of the daily diet has been found to lower levels of LDL, the so-called "bad" cholesterol.

Oil taken from wheat germ is also high in vitamin E. It can be ingested, or can be used externally to relieve sores or burns on the skin. Some research has suggested that octacosanol, an ingredient in wheat-germ oil, can help improve athletic performance and endurance. And some manufacturers have maintained that the presence of octacosanol makes wheat-germ oil a better source of vitamin E than other supplements, though such claims have been questioned by medical experts. While some early studies suggested that wheat-germ oil may have some beneficial effects in treating muscular dystrophy, more recent research disproved this theory.

Because it is such a good source of vitamin E, wheat germ may be helpful for many ailments and health conditions that appear to benefit from vitamin E supplementation.

PREPARATIONS

Available as flakes at grocery stores and health food stores. Also available in oil form. Wheat germ can become rancid, so it should be covered tightly and kept refrigerated.

TARGET AILMENTS

High LDL cholesterol

Heart disease

Cancer

Stroke

Diabetes

Fibrocystic breast disease

Menopausal symptoms

Other conditions that benefit from vitamin E supplementation

SIDE EFFECTS
NONE EXPECTED

ZINC

VITAL STATISTICS

GENERAL DESCRIPTION

The mineral zinc is integral to the synthesis of RNA and DNA, the genetic material that controls cell growth, division, and function. In various proteins, enzymes, hormones, and hormonelike substances called prostaglandins, zinc contributes to many bodily processes, including bone development and growth; cell respiration; energy metabolism; wound healing; the liver's ability to remove toxic substances such as alcohol from the body; immune function; and the regulation of heart rate and blood pressure. An adequate zinc intake enhances the ability to taste, promotes healthy skin and hair, enhances reproductive functions, and may improve short-term memory and attention span. As an anti-inflammatory agent, zinc is sometimes used to treat acne, rheumatoid arthritis, and prostatitis. Taking supplemental zinc may boost resistance to infection, especially in the elderly, and stimulate wound healing.

Many American diets are slightly low in zinc. Young children, pregnant women, vegetarians, and elderly people are most susceptible to zinc deficiency. Loss of taste is usually the first warning; other symptoms are hair loss or discoloration, white streaks on the nails, dermatitis, loss of appetite, fatigue, and poor wound healing.

Zinc ointment, which contains zinc oxide, is the most common topical form, useful in skin disorders, burns, and other wounds.

RDA
Adults: 15 mg
Pregnant women: 30 mg

NATURAL SOURCES
Zinc is most easily obtained from lean meat and seafood, but it is also found in eggs, soybeans, peanuts, wheat bran, cheese, oysters, and other foods.

PRECAUTIONS

☠ WARNING
Experts recommend increasing zinc levels by increasing the zinc-rich foods in your diet or by taking a multinutrient supplement that includes zinc chelate, zinc picolinate, or zinc aspartate, the three most easily absorbed forms. If zinc is used for more than three to six months to treat a chronic condition, it is essential to consult a nutritionist to avoid creating a mineral imbalance.

SPECIAL INFORMATION
- Zinc deficiency can retard growth in all children and stunt sexual development in boys.
- Ingesting extreme amounts of zinc daily can impair immune function and cause nausea, headaches, vomiting, dehydration, stomachaches, poor muscle coordination, fatigue, and possibly kidney failure.

TARGET AILMENTS
Immune problems

Skin problems

Wounds

SIDE EFFECTS
NONE EXPECTED

CONTINUED